POSITIVE PSYCHOLOGY
for Overcoming Depression

Also by Miriam Akhtar

The Happiness Training Plan CD,
www.happinesstrainingplan.com

POSITIVE PSYCHOLOGY

for Overcoming Depression

**Self-help strategies for
happiness, inner strength
and well-being**

MIRIAM AKHTAR, MAPP

WATKINS PUBLISHING
LONDON

*Dedicated to all those who have been visited
by the 'black dog' of depression*

This edition first published in the UK and USA 2012 by
Watkins Publishing, Sixth Floor, Castle House,
75–76 Wells Street, London W1T 3QH

Design and typography copyright © Paul Saunders 2012

Text copyright © Miriam Akhtar 2012

1 3 5 7 9 10 8 6 4 2

Designed and Typeset by Paul Saunders

Printed and bound in China by Imago

British Library Cataloguing-in-Publication Data Available
Library of Congress Cataloging-in-Publication Data Available

ISBN: 978-1-78028-104-9

www.watkinspublishing.co.uk

Distributed in the USA and Canada by Sterling Publishing Co., Inc.
387 Park Avenue South, New York, NY 10016-8810

For information about custom editions, special sales, premium and
corporate purchases, please contact Sterling Special Sales
Department at 800-805-5489 or specialsales@sterlingpub.com

Contents

Foreword

Medicine is far too obsessed with what makes us sick, and not nearly interested enough in what keeps us well. Working as a doctor is like camping beside a river. People float downstream and we dive deeper and deeper to pull out those who are sicker and sicker. And we're so busy and exhausted that no one has time to wander upstream and look at what's pushing people in. Depression is one of the biggest challenges facing us and the treatment desperately needs to move upstream. Everyone who's suffered from depression knows that tablets alone aren't the solution. But what is?

You will find the answer in this superb book. Positive psychology focuses on the science of what keeps us mentally healthy and happy. The beauty of this approach as both a treatment for, and preventative of depression, is that it's easy to understand, makes intuitive sense and – most importantly – there's solid scientific evidence to show that it works. It isn't happy-clappy psychobabble but is based on properly researched techniques and mindsets that can keep depression at bay.

In a nutshell, the research shows that if you focus on positive aspects of your life, this can reduce the negative emotions and feelings. I drag myself out of the doldrums with music, books, films, family and walks with the snout of a damp Labrador against my thigh. Modest pleasures, connecting with others and having a sense of meaning and purpose seem to keep me away from the Prozac. It was only when I read this book that I realized a lot of the things I instinctively do to stay positive have been proven to work and yet I rarely discuss them with patients. But I will now.

I've met lots of people with depression over the years, many of whom have been greatly helped by medication, at least in the short term, but all of whom are looking for ways to help themselves. As a family doctor, I have ten minutes (or six by the time the double-buggy is in and out the door) for each consultation and there's never enough time to go into any depth as to what might help my patient be happier and more resilient. This book, however, explores these questions in detail and with sensitivity and deserves to become a good friend to anyone who wants to improve their mental health. The question then is whether you can learn the benefits of positive psychology from a book, or whether you have to shell out for a happiness coach or therapist?

My advice is to give this book a go. If I was going to buy one book on positive psychology to treat depression, I'd choose an author who'd been properly trained as a positive psychologist, who knows how to write in an engaging and accessible way, and who understands, first-hand, the challenges of depression. In short, I'd choose Miriam. And if she went into every classroom in the country and taught children how to be resilient, happy and humane, I'd be pulling far fewer bodies out of the river later in life.

Dr Phil Hammond
Doctor, journalist, broadcaster and comedian
www.drphlhammond.com

Appreciation

I'd like to express my heart-felt gratitude to all those people who have contributed to the book. To Martin Seligman and all the researchers whose inspirational work I've cited. To my colleagues, friends and mentors in positive psychology; to the MAPP communities at the University of East London and the University of Pennsylvania and to all the clients and course participants that I've worked with. Special thanks go to the Fermé Park Road connection – Ann-Marie Evans for informally editing and to Sandra Rigby for formally editing. Thanks also to Ashley Akin-Smith, Bridget Grenville-Cleave, Paul Dodgson, Ilona Boniwell, Emma Judge, Fiona Parashar, Steve Humphries, Dr Chris Johnstone, Christina Robino, Pat Pilkington MBE, Fiona Dunlop, Elizabeth Digby-Firth, Fliss Barton, Denny Winstone, Ginette Ruthven, all at In-Volve, Jo Barnes and Molly Thompson for the many dog walks, and Shona Harris and Miranda Steed, for whom laughter is the best tonic whichever continent you're on. And finally to Archie and Oskar for reminding me what it's all about.

Preface

My story – how I discovered positive psychology

The insights in this book come from my professional practice as a positive psychologist and personal coach, my background in the media and as someone who spent a long time trying to overcome the 'black dog' of depression. Of all the relationships I've been in, one of the longest lasting was with depression. Mild, moderate or major – I've experienced them all. Now, it's rare for me to feel low and when I do dip down, I bounce back fast. I have learned how to keep the blues at bay – naturally – and developed my capacity for happiness.

Mine is not an unusual story. Every life has its ups and downs as I'm sure yours has too. Depression has a variety of causes, in my case what happened is that a pretty average childhood came to a sudden and brutal conclusion when my father collapsed and died. I was ten years old. Not long afterwards I went through the transition from junior to senior school. Life had changed radically in a short space of time and I felt the clouds gathering to block out the innocent sunshine of youth. I coped by becoming a teen workaholic. This was a successful strategy for many years and I did well in education and in my career. I had, though, a curious habit of interrupting positive experiences by asking myself 'But am I happy?' And in an instant the happiness would evaporate.

I had always imagined that by the Millennium I would be in a loving partnership with two children. But even though I went into my 30s in a relationship, a break-up led to me morphing into a singleton. Every birthday I wondered if this was the year that things would change, but there were already clues that family life might not be my fate. Just like Bridget Jones, the eponymous single girl, I had a creative job in an industry where over 50 percent of women aged 30+ do not have children. When you're married to the job it's very easy to miss out on the landmarks in life that we all take for granted, such as children. I took a sabbatical to deal with the Big Question that all singletons face. If I don't have children, then what am I going to do with my life?

Taking time out turned out to be a bad idea because it gave me too much space to dwell on what was wrong. Those grey clouds that had dogged me throughout life were gathering again. I usually suppressed them by throwing myself into yet another new project, but this time I spiralled downward. The doctor diagnosed depression and wrote a prescription for anti-depressants.

I ended up trying three types of anti-depressants, but none of them worked for me and their side-effects left me feeling worse. I went into therapy but all that did was put me in touch with my deepest pain. It didn't make me any happier. Talking about my long, dark night of the soul only served to keep me in that long, dark night. Like Bridget Jones I reached for the self-help books, but it felt like I was faking a happy smile to mask the undercurrent of despair.

What you focus on grows

The turning point came one morning when I noticed a funny smell coming from the dishwasher. Rank water was building up inside. Feeling bluer than blue, I thrashed around with some tools until a pipe burst and disaster – the kitchen flooded. Defeated I sat there on the damp floor and wailed. I'd spent months focusing on how *bad* I was feeling and where had it got me – to a sky-high bill for calling out the emergency plumber. I'd exhausted all the usual ways of dealing with depression, none of which were working for me. I was going to have to find my own road to recovery.

I'd first come across positive psychology in the mid-90s before its official birth as a new branch of psychology. I was intrigued to discover that there was a 'science' of happiness, that psychologists were applying the scientific method to investigate the characteristics of well-being in much the same way as it had been applied previously to study mental disorders and illness. It made a lot of sense to me. Here, at last, was evidence-based knowledge on how to develop our capacity for happiness. My interest was sparked initially by a radio programme I was producing on the subject, but over the next decade I applied my journalistic skills to investigate everything that was emerging from the new science of well-being. I devoured every book and research paper that I could get my hands on. Here was a goldmine of scientific knowledge that could make a substantial difference to human happiness.

Sitting there that day on the damp floor, I resolved to see how positive psychology might work for depression. So, out went the therapy and the pills and instead of focusing on how low I was feeling, I tried some of the techniques you'll find in this book. What happened was that slowly but surely I noticed the darkness began to recede and there were more and more days on which the sun came out from behind the clouds. I found a way out of depression and as a bonus discovered my purpose in life – to help others onto that path to happiness. I found what gives me meaning in life and the breakthrough had come courtesy of a broken dishwasher!

I wanted to share this knowledge, so I trained as a coach to put positive psychology into practice. Later Professor Martin Seligman, one of the co-founders of the science, established the Masters in Applied Positive Psychology (MAPP) at the University of Pennsylvania. The goal was to train the world's first positive psychologists:

'*Individuals whose practice will make the world a happier place, parallel to the way clinical psychologists have made the world a less unhappy place*'.[1] I completed the MAPP in the UK and became one of the first qualified positive psychologists in Europe. Now, I apply the science of well-being in my coaching practice and through my work as a trainer. Nothing gives me greater satisfaction than witnessing the change in people as their capacity for happiness grows and their lives begin to flourish. The positive changes on the inside are often matched by positive changes on the outside. Many of my clients fear, like I once did, that they might be incapable of happiness, so it is wonderful to see their pleasure and surprise when they discover that positive psychology really does work – they feel better and life takes a turn for the better.

I wish positive psychology had been around when I was that small girl who suffered a trauma. The well-being of young people is something that remains close to my heart. I work with organizations that help vulnerable youngsters and am one of the trainers of the Penn Resilience Programme,[2] which helps teenagers to build their resilience. Incidentally it's *never* too late to master the techniques of positive psychology, even if you have spent a lifetime in a relationship with depression. It just takes practice. It worked for me – I now enjoy a much more sustainable well-being – and it can work for you, too.

Miriam
www.positivepsychologytraining.co.uk

CHAPTER 1

The Positive Approach to Depression

IF YOU THINK YOU HAVE depression, you're not alone. It's one of the most widespread psychological disorders, so much so that it's often referred to as the common cold of mental health, although it's infinitely more distressing than a dose of the sniffles. We are living through a worldwide epidemic of depression – it's the number one threat to psychological well-being and the leading cause of disability in the 21st century. One in two adults in the developed world will experience an episode in their lifetime and having one incidence of depression raises the risk of future episodes. The average age at which people experience the first onset of depression has fallen from mid-life down to the early teens.

Wouldn't it be good to find something that inoculates against depression? Something that acts as protection against it just like putting on a thick jumper to keep out the cold? This is one of the ways in which positive psychology works for depression, by protecting you from it. It does this by building your resilience and well-being.

Positive psychology is a new branch of science. It's the scientific study of optimal functioning and well-being – how to feel good, function well and flourish. It goes under a number of aliases, such as the science of happiness, strengths, positive emotions, optimism and resilience, all of which give you an idea of the broad range of areas it covers.

Flourishing

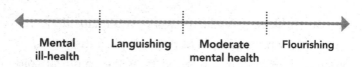

Mental ill-health   Languishing   Moderate mental health   Flourishing

The ultimate goal of positive psychology is to help you toward flourishing, a state of complete mental health, regardless of your starting point. If you have high emotional, psychological and social well-being, then you are flourishing. Languishing is where many people are. It is not quite illness but rather the absence of mental health, where life feels empty or hollow and you feel little positive emotion.

Since its inception in the late 1990s, positive psychology has developed evidence-based interventions that increase well-being. The techniques have been tried and tested in scientific studies, so we know that they work.

One of the beauties of positive psychology is that the strategies that build the positive have also been found to shrink the negative. So not only do positive psychology interventions raise happiness, but they also reduce the symptoms of depression.

DISEASE MODEL	**HEALTH MODEL**
Depression, Anxiety, Anger, Neurosis	Happiness, Well-being, Satisfaction, Joy
-10 ···················· 0	0 ···················· 10+
Repairing the worst in life	Building the best in life
Focus on weaknesses	Focus on strengths
Curing illness	Building well-being
Escaping unhappiness	Increasing happiness
Overcoming deficiencies	Developing competencies
Avoiding pain	Finding enjoyment
Zero as the ceiling	No ceiling

Positive psychology differs from most branches of psychology because it operates within the health model (the plus scale) rather than the disease model (the minus scale) used by clinicians and other mental health professionals. What this means is that the focus of positive psychology is on building what is good in life to increase well-being. Most types of therapy operate within the disease model where the emphasis is on repairing the worst in life to reduce suffering. This is the traditional approach to mental health, where the goal is to achieve an absence of mental illness or to reach zero or neutral, the border between illness and wellness, which you can see on the line in the chart (*see* page 3). So you're no longer suffering from a mental illness, but neither are you feeling good. You're left feeling empty rather than happy, languishing rather than flourishing. The point here is that the absence of depression is *not* the same as the presence of happiness, positive emotions or meaning in life. Positive psychology goes further, beyond the point of absence and into the presence of well-being. So the goal of the disease model is to get you from - to 0, whereas the goal of the health model is to get you from - past 0, and into +.

Most treatment for depression is based on the disease model and conventionally takes the form of antidepressant medication and/or psychotherapy. The positive psychology approach is different, with a goal of raising your level of well-being. You may wonder how this works in practice because what this does is put the focus on where you want to get to, rather than on what's ailing you. The input and effort goes into the goal you want to achieve, such as greater happiness, rather than on the issue of depression. As the saying goes, *'what you focus on is what you get'*. Focus on activities that promote happiness and the research indicates your happiness will grow. Coaching is the main tool used in positive psychology, a process that differs from the talking therapies on many levels.

Counselling	Coaching
• Focuses on the past	• Focuses on the future
• 'What is wrong?'	• 'What do you want?'
• Emotional understanding	• Behavioural mentoring
• Looks at pain and difficulty	• Sets goals
• Release from the past	• Moving forward

Counselling aims to facilitate an emotional understanding of the problem in the hope that the insights you gain in the session will lead to a cathartic release from pain. This may serve a purpose in coming to terms with the cause of depression, but there is also the risk with talking about your unhappiness that you can end up drowning in that very unhappiness – that you get stuck in the pain rather than moving past it.

Psychotherapy became widely accepted as the therapy of choice for depression during the 20th century. It is based on a bold (but largely untested) truism: that talking about your troubles will lead to a cure.[1] Research indicates that the positive changes that occur in therapy are more likely to be the result of the relationship with the therapist than the form of therapy practised.[2] Psychotherapy is not for everyone – some research has shown that it can lead to a worsening of symptoms in around 10 percent of cases.[3] My own experience of therapy was that it led to reviving rather than resolving the emotional pain I was suffering. What the therapeutic process seems to lack is a strategy of building the positives to replace the considerable negatives of depression.

So, what if you've had enough of being immersed in what's wrong and want to focus on regaining well-being? This is where positive psychology comes in. Its techniques are designed to encourage positive emotions, thoughts and behaviour and by doing this they also have the delightful consequence of reducing depressive symptoms. By focusing on the positive, you can also alleviate the negative.

I've seen this work many a time with coaching clients, who experience 'aha' moments when they suddenly realize that they no longer feel as gloomy as they once did. Happiness has crept up on them and it's all happened naturally. One of my most memorable experiences of this was when I ran a pilot of positive psychology for vulnerable adolescents with alcohol problems.[4] They drank to escape from their problems, as a shortcut to get happy and as a quick release from the stress they felt. These young people lacked stability in their lives – most were in temporary accommodation, estranged from their families, living in hostels or 'sofa-surfing'. They were dealing with all kinds of problems – abuse, violence, drugs, crime, family breakdown, ill-health, bereavement, literacy and financial difficulties. Virtually all had dropped out of education, some were young offenders with tags on their ankles and there was one pregnant teenager. None of them had any faith in the future.

Instead of taking the approach of focusing on their alcohol problems as per normal 'disease model' treatment, those issues were put to one side with only one out of the 16 hours of the programme directly addressing their binge-drinking. Instead, the course concentrated on well-being with sessions on happiness, positive emotions, optimism, resilience, meditation, strengths, positive relationships, goal-setting and the body-mind connection.

This turned out to be a spectacularly successful approach. As the weeks went by the young people started feeling better and began to flourish. The positive changes that were happening on the inside were mirrored by an abundance of positive consequences on the outside. Most of the group returned to education, some got new jobs and new accommodation, relationships were repaired, there was calm in place of the usual chaos and a visible improvement in their vitality. It amounted to a transformation. The most exciting side-effect of this focus on well-being was that drinking dropped dramatically – by two-thirds – with some giving up alcohol altogether. And this was achieved by parking those alcohol problems! Incidentally, the pregnant teenager, who was so pessimistic that her key worker described her as 'almost afraid to think of what good can happen for fear of what bad might happen', went on to give birth to a baby daughter and named her ... Faith.

This gives you some idea of the effectiveness of operating in the health model, where the effort is put into the goal rather than the issue. These positive results echo the findings of the first scientific survey of positive psychology interventions, a meta-analysis combining statistical results from thousands of study participants, which showed that not only do these techniques significantly increase happiness, but they work even better on depression symptoms.[5] One of the interventions in the analysis was Positive Psychotherapy, which contrasts with standard treatment for depression by focusing on increasing positive emotion, strengths and meaning in life rather than directly targeting the symptoms of depression. Positive Psychotherapy was tested on people with mild-to-moderate depression where it was found to significantly decrease levels of depression. It has also been tested on severely depressed individuals as a supplement to traditional treatment methods, where it relieved the symptoms of depression and led to more remission than either drug treatment or 'treatment as usual'.[6] These studies show that positive psychology has a valuable role to play in broadening the choices of treatment for depression.

Turning to you ...

So you're depressed. Or you think you may be heading that way. It could be that you've been down for a while and are looking for a new way of dealing with it. Or maybe you sense depression creeping up on you and want to stop it in its tracks? Positive psychology techniques can be used as a natural way to lift your mood, to protect you from depression and to complement other forms of treatment.

It's normal to sometimes feel down, sad or unhappy, usually in reaction to a particular event such as an ending, a disappointment or something going wrong. This is part of life's ups and downs and people usually recover. Depression, however, goes beyond that to intense feelings of sadness, negativity, anxiety and hopelessness. The difference is that these emotions persist in depression and interfere with day-to-day activities.

Depression compromises your well-being and reduces your quality of life. It affects how you feel on the inside and how life happens on the outside. The world has a grey, leaden feel to it that weighs on the body, turns the mind negative, drives the emotions down and saps the spirit. Living with depression is fraught with problems, not only for you, but also for your loved ones. As well as not feeling good, it can compromise your ability to function in your life and impact on relationships.

So how do you know if you are experiencing depression? It could be that you've lost interest in the things you used to enjoy. Maybe you've been feeling sad, anxious, overwhelmed, pessimistic or in despair. Physically you may be exhausted, tearful and lethargic. You may be withdrawing from loved ones and minimizing your contact with the world. Any and all of these are symptoms of depression. You may not even recognize that you're depressed. Many of us don't. It can take someone else to point out that you haven't been your usual self for a while and to ask what's wrong. Sometimes it's only when the doctor hands you the diagnosis that you realise what you've been suffering. Of the many symptoms of depression, probably the most widely recognized is a persistent low mood and a marked loss of interest in life. If it is causing you distress, affecting your normal functioning, there are other symptoms present and this has been going on for more than two weeks, then this is the gauge that doctors generally use to diagnose depression. Scan this list to see how many of these items apply to you on a regular or continuing basis.

Psychological symptoms include:
- persistent low mood or sadness
- marked loss of interest or enjoyment in activities
- feelings of hopelessness and helplessness
- poor concentration
- low self-esteem, feeling worthless
- feeling anxious or worried
- excessive or inappropriate guilt
- feeling irritable and intolerant of others
- lack of motivation
- indecisiveness, difficulty making decisions
- recurring thoughts of death
- suicidal thoughts or thoughts of harming yourself

→

Physical symptoms include:

- tiredness, exhaustion, lack of energy
- tearfulness
- disturbed sleep patterns
- unexplained aches and pains
- slowed movement/speech or restlessness/agitation
- change in appetite; weight gain or loss
- digestive problems
- reduced sex drive
- changes to the menstrual cycle

Social symptoms include:

- difficulties in home and family life
- work performance suffering
- avoiding contact with friends
- taking part in fewer social activities
- reduced interests

What causes depression?

People develop depression for all kinds of reasons. It is a complex disorder with multiple causes and consequences for your mood, thoughts and body. It's also common for people to blame themselves for developing depression.

Thoughts like 'I'm no good' or 'I wish I could be more like ...' or 'if only I could do ...' are assumed to be at the root of the depression when they are more likely to be symptoms of it. It is useful to understand what factors in your life may have contributed to the downward spiral into depression. Mental health professionals typically group the risk factors for depression into three categories, the 3 Ps.[7]

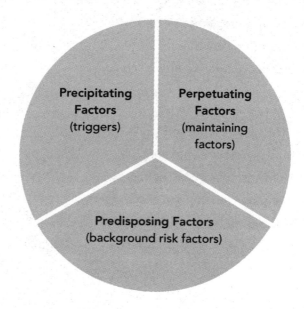

Precipitating Factors (triggers)

Perpetuating Factors (maintaining factors)

Predisposing Factors (background risk factors)

Predisposing factors are the features of your background that increase your risk to depression. This includes your genes, upbringing, personal history, culture, recent events, your health, diet and other factors. Some of these you can change and others you have no control over.

Precipitating factors are the psychological and physical triggers that can tip you over into depression, such as stress, illness or trauma.

Perpetuating factors differ from the other two causes by being things that happen *afterwards*. An example of this is drinking heavily as a way of coping with depression. The chemical effect of alcohol on the brain is also a cause of depression. This can set up a vicious cycle where the more depressed you feel, the more you drink, which in turn leads to feeling even more depressed.

Positive psychology has its own 3 Ps of depression in the way that pessimists explain negative events to themselves. When a bad thing happens to pessimists, they tend to think that it's **personal** ('it's all my fault'), **permanent** ('it can't change') and **pervasive** ('it'll affect everything). Pessimism is a thinking style that puts you on the fast track to depression. Here are some of the other factors that can contribute to depression.[8]

Stressful life events

Relationship breakdowns, bereavement, redundancy – it takes time to adjust to traumatic events. Your risk of becoming depressed is increased if you stop seeing friends and family and try to deal with problems on your own.

Physical illness

You have a higher risk of depression if you have a chronic health condition or a life-threatening illness. Depression is a common consequence of pain and illness. If you suffer insomnia, you're also at risk.

Personality

Certain character traits can make you more vulnerable to depression, such as being perfectionist, overly self-critical, pessimistic, prone to excessive worrying, having a rigid thinking style, low self-esteem or little sense of control over life.

Family history

If either of your parents experienced depression, then you're at a higher risk of developing it yourself. Certain genes increase the likelihood of depression after a stressful life event.

Isolation

Living an isolated life, cut off from others, can increase your risk of loneliness and depression. Having an active social life is one of the characteristics of the world's happiest people.

Alcohol and drugs

There is a relationship between substance use and depression. Alcohol and drugs are often used to cope with stress and depression, but the sad truth is that they can also lead to depression.

Being female

Women are almost twice as likely as men to experience depression. One of the reasons for this is the hormonal fluctuations of the menstrual cycle, in particular during the perimenopause (mid-30s to 40s), but also as a result of pregnancy, infertility, the menopause and, in some women, childlessness. One compensation is that as well as experiencing lower lows, women also tend to have higher highs of happiness than men.

The degrees of depression

Depression comes in a variety of forms and grades of severity from mild to moderate and major. Some forms of depression are chronic whereas others are episodic, with an average episode lasting for between six and eight months.

✦ At the milder end of the disorder is sub-clinical depression, which has some impact on your daily life. The treatment is generally based on guided self-help, lifestyle changes such as regular exercise and/or some form of therapy or group support.

✦ With moderate depression there are more symptoms present and it has a significant impact on your daily life. Additional treatment options include the talking therapies – counselling, psychotherapy or CBT (Cognitive-Behavioural Therapy).

✦ Major depressive disorder or clinical depression is at the severe end. You have many of the symptoms, which have a pronounced effect on your functioning, making the activities of daily life near impossible. Anti-depressant medication is a likely treatment, which can be complemented with other options.

✦ Dysthymia is a form of clinical depression. This is a low grade, mild depression, which can last for years and for this reason is often treated with medication.

✦ Bi-polar disorder is characterized by a cycle of manic highs, hypomania, alternating with the sometimes more frequent lows of major depressive episodes. Cyclothymia is a milder version of bi-polar disorder.

✦ The hormonal and physical changes after giving birth, added to the responsibility for a new life, can lead to postnatal depression.

✦ SAD – Seasonal Affective Disorder is the 'winter blues' where the absence of daylight as winter approaches leads to a plummeting mood.

The downward spiral

Depression is a downward spiral that operates in a variety of programmes – a bit like computer software. See if you recognize the version you might be experiencing.

Version 1.0 The thought/emotion spiral

You're having negative thoughts that send your emotions plummeting, which in turn makes your thoughts even bleaker and your mood then spirals down to an even lower place.

Version 1.1 The social spiral

Another one goes like this. You feel down so you don't feel up to seeing people and, because you don't reach out, there's no distraction from your low mood and you sink even lower.

Version 1.2 The physical spiral

This is a variation on 1.1 – you're exhausted; your body hurts, which depresses your mood; you can't summon the energy to do anything physical and, again, your mood sinks lower.

Version 1.3 The pessimistic spiral

One of the downward spirals specifically targeted by positive psychology runs like this. You expect the worst to happen, that a situation is out of your control, over-whelming and doomed to failure. That in itself leaves you down. The situation needs sorting, but because you don't believe you can make a difference to the outcome, you don't put in the effort to make it work. Instead, you give up. Your mood sinks even lower into despair. This is the cycle of 'learned helplessness', which feeds depression.

Many of these spirals act like computer viruses – they spread and merge. So, for example, you may have been down because you were ill (physical), which stops you seeing people (social) and you then feel pessimistic about things ever getting better (psychological), which sends your mood down into depression.

Using this book

This book offers a positive approach to depression with self-help strategies for mild or chronic forms of unhappiness. Research has shown that this positive approach works well in reducing the symptoms of depression. If you suffer from low moods or the milder end of depression and are looking for a natural way of boosting your mood, then these techniques can help. If you're experiencing a more severe form of depression, you should consult a physician for their advice. The tools can be used in conjunction with other forms of treatment or to consolidate your recovery. All the strategies are scientifically grounded, based on evidence from positive psychology research. Instead of focusing on exploring what's wrong in the hope that fresh understanding will reduce unhappiness, they directly target happiness and well-being. The first part of the book tells you what you need to know about the science of happiness, well-being and positive emotions, and the self-help strategies begin in Chapter 4 with Savouring, one of the core positive psychology techniques, and continue to the final chapter. Each of these chapters also refers you to key texts from positive psychology for further reading on the strategies.

What are the tools for?

✦ To boost mood naturally

✦ To protect from depression

✦ To overcome mild depression and chronic low mood

✦ To increase happiness and well-being

✦ As a supplement to depression treatment

✦ To prevent relapse into depression

✦ To relieve the residual symptoms of major depression

Depression – a third way

Depression affects your feelings, thoughts and body, with each of these three dimensions impacting on the others. It's a disorder of mind, body and spirit and this is reflected in the chapters that follow. Approach your self-management of depression by considering strategies on every level – emotional, cognitive, physical, social and your direction in life.

It would be unrealistic to imagine that you can make the transition from depression to happiness in one big leap. What's more, happiness is not a permanent state. Those top-of-the-range emotions like bliss, elation and ecstasy are passing experiences even outside of depression. The goal here is not so much to chase those momentary highs, but rather to invest in raising your underlying, or what could be called 'constant' level of contentment – a more realistic prospect. This is a far more sustainable form of happiness. So, aim to do things that leave you feeling a bit better on a regular basis.

A user's guide

There is a saying in coaching: 'If you do what you've always done, you'll get what you've always got.' This book offers a new and different approach to depression, based on increasing positivity. For some people this will seem counter-intuitive and far too indirect – why mess around with happiness techniques when the problem is depression? However, remember that depression shrinks your view of your capabilities and keeps you in a comfort zone of lowness. This is about trying something different, because if you do what you've always done, you'll get what you've always got. One of the other principles of coaching is that the answer lies within you, the client. You are the best guide as to what will work well for you, so trust your instincts. You are more likely to persist with a technique if you are drawn to it. Here are some other tips on using positive psychology techniques in depression.

1. Adopt a 'growth mindset'

Do you have a fixed or a growth mindset? Do you believe that your abilities are more or less set in stone or that you can become better at most things with enough effort and motivation? According to psychologist Carol Dweck, author of *Mindset*,[9] these are the two mindsets that govern our behaviour and influence our ability to develop and grow.

A **fixed mindset** is where you believe that you were born with a certain set of talents – born clever, sporty, creative, good with numbers, good with people, etc – and that those capabilities are more or less fixed at birth. So, if something goes wrong – such as the breakdown of a relationship – it's taken as proof that you're not as good at relationships as you believed yourself to be and this can lead to a loss of self-confidence. A fixed mindset person is less likely to put in the effort to develop their capabilities and more likely to stop trying and feel depressed when they fail to make the grade (in their eyes).

The **growth mindset** has a different starting point, viewing people as more malleable and with a huge potential for growth and development. With enough motivation, effort and concentration we can become better at almost anything. People who have a growth mindset don't take failure so personally. They see it more as feedback that will help them to improve their performance next time around. They're more likely to be flexible and try following other routes to get to their goal. So they don't give up, instead they learn and develop.

Positive psychology operates in a 'growth mindset' with a belief that things are more flexible than they are fixed, that we can learn optimism, grow our capacity for happiness and develop our strengths. So, adopt a 'growth mindset' when trying out the techniques. Have a go and if something doesn't work first time, remember that this is feedback to be flexible – try a different approach or have another go later.

2. Just one thing a day

Depression is a profoundly energy-sapping experience and it can be very hard to get motivated to do anything. That's why my advice is to think in baby steps and aim to do just one small thing a day – a nudge in the right direction. Be kind to yourself. Of course, you can always do more than that, but don't beat yourself up if it turns out to be unsustainable. Think small.

3. Know who you are

Think of how you are when you're not down in the dumps. So, if you're normally quite sociable, you might invest in nurturing your relationships or engaging in a social activity. Variety is the spice of life for some so, if you get bored easily, come up with your own twist on a technique to keep it fresh or make it a better fit for you.

4. Go for a stretch

Be experimental, too, by trying something new. Go for a stretch and venture out of your comfort zone.

✦ If you're very much 'in your head', you might try one of the physical strategies in Vitality (Chapter 10).

✦ If your tendency is to be overly analytical, try one of the Positive Emotions techniques (Chapter 3).

✦ If your emotions are overwhelming, look at some of the exercises in Positive Directions (Chapter 12) to focus your attention onto something practical.

✦ And if your instinct normally is to leap straight into action, how about slowing down and addressing your thinking habits in Learning Optimism (Chapter 7).

5. Persistence and patience

Some of these techniques work by training the mind to notice what's good in life and get over the brain's negativity bias, which draws attention to what's wrong. This requires persistence and patience – it takes 21 days of repeats to acquire a habit. But gradually, like a dimmer switch, the light will come on and your experience of happiness and positive emotions will grow.

Enjoy the journey!

CHAPTER 2

The Positive Psychology Story of Happiness

BEFORE WE DELVE INTO the techniques themselves, I'd like to share with you some of the story of positive psychology as the scientific study of happiness and a few of the theories it has generated. This will give you some clues as to what you might be missing from your well-being. Psychology had three broad aims in the first half of the 20th century – to cure mental illness, to nurture high talent and to improve people's lives. But after the trauma of the Second World War the science narrowed its scope into identifying and treating mental illness. This led to great progress being made in alleviating the suffering caused by mental disorder, but what it meant was that the positive aspects of life – such as investigating what it takes for us to flourish – became neglected areas of research. Instead, psychology began to view people more as passive victims of their internal pathological drives, damaged brains or external stressors. We were left with an unbalanced science which had become a psychology of the negative, focusing most of its research into what is wrong and weak in people, highlighting shortcomings over strengths.

Positive psychology emerged as a new branch of science in the late 1990s as an attempt to rebalance the field and apply the scientific method to questions such as what it takes for us to feel good and function well. This has led to an abundance of research in areas of well-being, such as happiness, positive emotions, strengths, optimism, hope, flow, mindfulness, love, wisdom, courage, creativity, authenticity, motivation and goals. The science has built on the foundations of its predecessor, humanistic psychology, which similarly avoided the what-is-wrong-with-people approach to focus instead on human potential, growth, fulfilment and self-actualization. Although it has the positive tag, this doesn't mean that the science of well-being doesn't 'do' negative or that it ignores or denies the difficult aspects of life. In fact there is one area of the science – post-traumatic growth – which is about life's major crises and the unexpected gains that can emerge from shattering events. Positive psychology deals with the negative in the main by looking at positive ways of coping and through exploring areas such as resilience – how to bounce back from life's tough times and thrive in periods of adversity.

This branch of psychology was co-founded by Professor Martin Seligman, author of *Learned Optimism* and *Authentic Happiness*, alongside Professor Mihaly Csikszentmihalyi, who put the study of 'flow' on the map. Seligman's own career has paralleled the transition in psychology from studying the negative to the positive, from 'learned help-lessness' to 'learned optimism'. At the heart of the field is the study of 'subjective well-being', the scientific term for happiness that reflects the personal way in which we rate our well-being. We now know a lot more about the anatomy of happiness, what it is and how to achieve it. Scientists have come up with a number of formulae, some of which are discussed below. The research will also give you clues as to what might be involved in your downward spiral into depression. But first the good news ...

The 40 percent equation

A big fat 40 percent of your happiness is under your direct voluntary control and can be increased by the activities you engage in and your outlook on life.[1] So, regardless of the hand you've been dealt in life, there is a lot you can do to influence your level of happiness.

$$H = S + C + V^2$$

H is your enduring level of happiness. Think of it as your constant level of contentment rather than being about momentary positive emotions such as joy.

S is your set range of happiness. This is determined by your genes and accounts for around 50 percent of

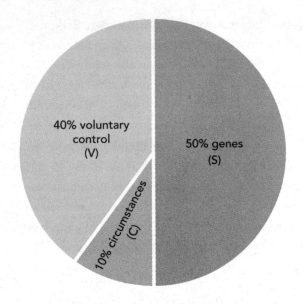

happiness. Whether you have a significant positive or negative life experience, you will eventually revert to your set range.

C is for your circumstances or conditions of your life. This accounts for only 10 percent of your happiness, which is probably less than you might imagine. So, changing your circumstances, such as going for a better job or moving to a new house, will only have a marginal effect on your happiness.

V is the bit that's under your voluntary control and that accounts for around 40 percent of your happiness. So nearly half of our happiness can be influenced by engaging in voluntary activities such as the positive psychology techniques described in this book.

Happiness is ...

Martin Seligman identified three main pathways to authentic happiness,[3] which will help you work out where you seek yours and what, if anything, might be out of balance.

Pleasure is about the feel-good factor, enjoyment, positive emotions and energy.

Engagement is about the depth of your involvement with life – with work, people, activities. It also refers to 'flow' (more on which later).

Meaning is about the things that give your life meaning and purpose.

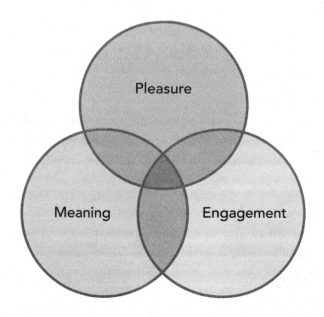

PERMA[4]

The pleasure - engagement - meaning model of happiness was upgraded in 2011 to PERMA, a theory of well-being that is broader than happiness. Each of these pathways to well-being is featured in this book.

✦ Positive emotion

✦ Engagement

✦ Relationships

✦ Meaning

✦ Achievement

> SWB (subjective well-being) =
> SWL + high PA + low NA[5]

This formula for subjective well-being combines how you think about happiness (cognitive) with how you feel about it (emotional).

SWL stands for 'satisfaction with life'. This is how you rate your life compared to your ideal of how life should be. So, if there is a discrepancy between where you are now and your ideal, you'll be low on life satisfaction.

PA (high) stands for Positive Affect and refers to your experience of positive emotions. This is more about the frequency with which you experience positive emotions rather than the intensity.

NA (low) is the opposite, it stands for Negative Affect, the sum of your experience of negative emotions. Subjective well-being requires the quantity of positive affect to be higher than negative affect.

Psychological well-being[6]

There are six elements in this model of well-being. If you can put a tick in each of these categories, then you are likely to be experiencing psychological well-being. If you are low in any of these domains, then that is a clue as to where you can apply your focus.

✦ Self-acceptance – accepting yourself for who you are

✦ Positive relationships – having quality connections to others

✦ Life purpose – having meaningful goals and direction in life

✦ Personal growth – fostering ongoing growth and personal development

✦ Autonomy – having a sense of personal control in thought and action

✦ Environmental mastery – managing your life and surroundings effectively

Flow[7]

Flow is a different type of happiness, a state of absorption where you're fully immersed in a pleasing activity, such that you may lose track of time. Flow is about being totally engaged with what you're doing – in the moment or in the zone – and it's generally after, rather than during, the experience that you appreciate the pleasure it brings. The process itself is sometimes characterized by a lack of emotion. What puts you into flow is very individual and is often related to your personal interests, whether creative, sporty, vocational, educational or spiritual. Reading, dancing, gardening, making music, jogging and cookery are often mentioned as flow-inducers. A friend of mine goes into flow playing with her grandson's model railways!

Self-determination theory[8]

This formula suggests that we have three fundamental needs that have to be met in order to have well-being.

✦ **Autonomy** – having a sense of control over what you do

✦ **Competence** – feeling confident in what you do

✦ **Relatedness** – having close, secure connections to people

Short high or sustainable happiness?

By now you'll have realized that there is more than one form of happiness or well-being and an abundance of routes to it (thankfully!) They can be divided into one of two types.

+ **Hedonic well-being** is the instantly recognizable form of happiness. This is the 'high' of happiness from pleasure and positive emotions such as love. It's an intense form of happiness, strongly related to a cheerful mood.

+ **Eudaimonic well-being** (*see* page 221) is the second form of happiness, based on the ancient Greek term 'daimon', which refers to your true nature. This is about how you are when you're at your best, when you're realizing your potential. It is related to the things that give your life meaning and is a deeper, more enduring form of well-being.

A happy balance

It's good to recognize which form of happiness works well for you or which you'd like more of. Let's consider Seligman's three pathways to authentic happiness. Pleasure is a hedonic form of happiness which generates a short-term high that is concentrated but fades fast. That's because we have a 'hedonic treadmill'; we adapt to the things that give us pleasure and begin to take them for granted so they stop working as well. The vanilla cupcake is never as scrumptious the second time around. After a while your new car fails to give you the thrill it did when you first drove it home. Engagement and Meaning, on the other hand, are both eudaimonic forms of well-being – there are fewer good feelings, but engaging and meaningful activities can lead to a greater satisfaction with life over the long term.

Your life map

Have a go at looking at your own life and noting your balance between Pleasure, Engagement and Meaning. Choose a time span, maybe the last 24 hours or the last week. How did you spend your time? Think back over your activities and list them in the left-hand column. Then decide which category, if any, they fall into – Pleasure, Engagement (Flow) or Meaning.

Ask yourself these questions:

✦ What is the balance like between the three main columns?

✦ Is the balance how you would like it to be?

✦ Do you need more, less or the same amount of time for each column?

✦ What three actions could you take to achieve a better balance?

ACTIVITY	TYPE OF HAPPINESS			
	Pleasure	Engagement (Flow)	Meaning	None of these

By doing this you'll begin to get a sense of whether the balance in your life is toward the short high of hedonic well-being or the deeper fulfilment of eudaimonic well-being, and whether this is right for you or not.

The facts and fiction of happiness

While we're talking about the pursuit of happiness, let's bust some of the myths that can hold us back in our quest for personal contentment. Here's the lowdown on what the science tells us about what does and doesn't make us happy.

Makes us happy?	Fact	Fiction
Wealth		✘ Once there's enough money to cover the necessities of life, money ceases to have much impact on our well-being.
Love and Connections	✔ Relationships and being actively social are major sources of happiness.	
Education		✘ Your level of education has little impact on happiness.

→

Makes us happy?	Fact	Fiction
Work	✔ Engaging work and job satisfaction count.	
Youth		✘ Happiness does not decline with age. There is a low point around the mid-40s but then it rises again.
Physical well-being	✔ Sleep, exercise and food affect your mood.	
Beauty		✘ Being physically attractive does not mean greater happiness.
Spirituality	✔ Engaging in some form of religious practice has benefits.	
Living in a sunny climate		✘ Sunshine and warmth only have a marginal effect on your happiness.
Health	✔ What you think about your state of health has an impact ...	✘ ... but the reality of your health has little connection to your level of happiness, except in the case of serious illness.

→

Makes us happy?	Fact	Fiction
Children	✔ Having children can give your life meaning…	✗… but doesn't make you any happier, especially where the toddler and teen years are concerned.

PS on the pursuit of happiness

For such a desirable goal (happiness is enshrined in the American Constitution as a human right), pursuing it is a haphazard affair. In my personal experience I've found that making happiness the direct goal is more likely to backfire, as it slips in and out of your hands. To paraphrase John Lennon, happiness seems to happen while you're busy making other plans. Happiness is best regarded as a by-product of your attempts to raise your general well-being. There is some evidence to suggest that when you set happiness itself as the goal, you're likely to have unrealistically high standards and to be disappointed when you fail to reach those heights or stay up there.[9] It is far better to set a low goal – aim for a feeling of contentment rather than the high of happiness. As many positive psychology models suggest, there is a lot more to happiness than feeling good. Engage fully with positive moments as and when they occur – savour them, but suspend any heavy analysis of whether you're feeling happier or not. Keep a light touch about raising your level of happiness and remember that those peak moments are ephemeral. Enjoy them in the moment, but don't cling onto them. And remember that the pursuit of happiness is much broader than the pursuit of pleasure. There are all those activities that bring meaning, purpose and engagement into life.

In the next chapter we look at one of the major players in the recovery from depression – positive emotions – with the chapters that follow exploring the techniques that will raise your experience of them.

Resources
Authentic Happiness and Flourish, both by Martin Seligman
Flow by Mihaly Csikszentmihalyi
The HOW of Happiness by Sonja Lyubomirsky
Positive Psychology in a Nutshell by Ilona Boniwell
The Happiness Training Plan CD by Dr Chris Johnstone & Miriam Akhtar (www.happinesstrainingplan.com)
Positive Psychology News Daily (www.positivepsychologynews.com)
Positive Psychology (UK) (www.positivepsychology.org.uk)

CHAPTER 3

Positive Emotions: The Upward Spiral to Well-being

✦ **What is it?** Positive emotions are the key to the positive approach to depression

✦ **In other words:** Positive emotions not only feel good, they do us good, too

✦ **Try this for:** Boosting mood naturally, happiness, resilience and well-being

joy, love, awe, inspiration, excitement, ecstasy, bliss, amusement, creativity, gratitude, contentment, calm, serenity, satisfaction, peace, hope, trust ...

Ah, the joy of positive emotions ... so delightful when they arise and yet so elusive in depression! They might bubble up through that loving connection you have with someone or in that quiet space of peace and satisfaction; when you are inspired by a new idea or awestruck by the beauty of nature. Positive emotions may be fleeting, but these good feelings play a vital role in well-being and the recovery from depression. There is a power in positive emotions that goes beyond the pleasure in the moment. One of the main discoveries in positive psychology has been that positive emotions not only feel good, they do us good, too. They help us to feel better, to recover from adversity and to access an upward spiral of emotional well-being, which counteracts the downward spiral into depression, and they also bolster us against life's stresses.

Positive emotions hold the key to the positive psy-chology approach to depression. I experienced how well this works in my own journey out of depression. I spent years exploring my negative emotions in therapy, dig-ging deep into my unhappiness, each time re-opening the wounds and bringing past hurt to the front of my mind. But it wasn't until I went down the opposite route, that of boosting positive emotions that I finally began to recover and move out of depression. You'll find many of the techniques that build positive emotions in the chapters that follow.

The role of emotions

Emotions are part of being human and reflect the complexity of human nature. You can experience both positive and negative emotions at the same time – joy tinged with sadness, for example. Emotions tend to be short-lived and focused on something specific whereas moods are longer-lasting and are more free-floating rather than being the consequence of something.

In their simplest form, our emotions act as signals. A negative emotion, such as fear or anger, tells us that something is wrong and needs fixing, whereas a positive emotion lets us know that something good is happening and we're on track toward our hopes and goals.

Negative emotions alert us to danger, sending out a warning that something needs to be sorted out – and quickly. These emotions prompt us into specific actions. They served an evolutionary purpose in activating the survival instincts of our ancestors. Anger leads to attack, fear to escape. The prehistoric family, faced with a large mammal charging toward them, would experience fear, prompting them to flee. The same still holds true today. Faced with a runaway car hurtling toward you, you will be propelled by fear to get out of the way. Negative emotions narrow our thinking, so that we can tackle the immediate threat to our well-being. They are powerful experiences.

I remember the day I moved into a room above a café, when I was a student living in France. My neighbour seemed friendly and showed me around the place. Late that night there was a knock at the door. I opened it and to my horror the neighbour was standing there wearing nothing but his birthday suit ... ! In that moment of sheer terror, I managed to shove a heavy wardrobe across the door. I trembled all night until I heard the café owner arrive in the morning to open up downstairs. It was then that I went to move the wardrobe. Only I found it really hard to shift, whereas during the night the emotion of fear had given me the presence of mind and strength to spot the wardrobe's potential to shield me and move it in a flash. This illustrates how negative emotions can work for us. They narrow our thought–action repertoires to those that best suit our survival in threatening situations.

Negative emotions like fear and anxiety are generally much 'louder' experiences than positive emotions, even when there is no immediate threat involved. They also last longer – they hang around and weigh you down, whereas positive emotions are much lighter, more fleeting experiences. In the past, psychology research was largely focused on studying negative emotions and not much was known about the purpose of those short-lived, positive experiences. That was until Barbara Fredrickson emerged as the world's leading researcher on positive emotions.

What positive emotions can do for you

Barbara Fredrickson discovered that there are benefits to experiencing positive emotions that go far beyond the short-lived good feeling. The effects of positivity are subtle but substantial. Positive emotions open up our hearts and minds. They nourish us. Whereas negative emotions narrow and focus our thinking, positive emotions broaden our thinking and over time accumulate to build multiple resources that support our well-being. Fredrickson named this the broaden-and-build theory of positive emotions.[1]

POSITIVE EMOTIONS

Past	Present	Future
Contentment	Love	Hope
Satisfaction	Awe	Optimism
Fulfilment	Joy	Faith
Pride	Bliss	Trust
Serenity	Ecstasy	
Gratitude	Inspiration	
	Calm	
	Peace	
	Pleasure	
	Curiosity	
	Interest	
	Excitement	
	Amusement	
	Open	
	Creativity	

Broaden the mind

Positive emotions broaden our thinking, the scope of our attention and prompt us into a wide range of action. They make us more open-minded, creative and flexible thinkers, capable of envisioning the big picture. If you want to generate some new ideas or find a creative answer, you might be better off doing something that makes you feel good rather than stressing your way to the solution. Positive emotions broaden our thought–action repertoires.

◆ **Joy** leads to an urge to play, to push the limits and to be creative.

◆ **Interest** causes a desire to seek out new information, to explore the world and to expand the self.

◆ **Contentment** is a prompt to savour and integrate new perspectives into your world.

◆ **Pride** makes you think big.

◆ **Elevation** inspires you to become better.

◆ **Love** makes you want to share and explore with others, plus all of the above.

Build up resources

Positive emotions are the gifts that keep on giving! Although short-lived in themselves, they accumulate to produce long-lasting personal resources that we can draw on at other times.

✦ **Psychological resources** Positive emotions help to develop optimism and resilience. They also shape your sense of identity and stimulate the motivation to pursue goals.

✦ **Intellectual resources** Positive emotions boost problem-solving skills and assist with learning new information.

✦ **Social resources** Positive emotions help you in forming new relationships and solidify the bonds of existing ones.

✦ **Physical resources** Positive emotions help you develop co-ordination, strength and cardiovascular health.

Some of these benefits, such as positive emotions building physical resources, may surprise you. However, if you're feeling curious, for example, you're more likely to explore the world around you and this, in turn, leads to physical activity, which builds muscle, fitness, etc.

Speed recovery from negative emotions

If you're suffering from stress positive emotions are particularly relevant. Experiments have revealed how positive emotions can undo the ill effects that negativity has on the body, such as increasing blood pressure and raising heart rate, and help it return to homeostasis, a state of equilibrium. A feeling of contentment or amusement, for example, speeds the physical recovery from stress. Barbara Fredrickson calls this your 'hidden reset button'.

You can't stop your heart from beating harder when faced with stress, but positivity will help to rein in those cardiovascular reactions and regain a calm heart.[2] In her experiments Fredrickson showed film clips that evoked positive emotions such as serenity and amusement, which led to people recovering faster from the after-effects of negativity than when they were shown negative or neutral clips. This is something you can easily adapt for yourself when you experience negativity – watch a comedy, for instance, or listen to some calming or uplifting music.

Positive emotions protect you from depression and can stop you relapsing. The more positivity you experience, the greater is your ability to cope with adversity because the broadened thinking that positivity produces enables you to spot more solutions to the problem. Positivity builds your resilience. It's like filling a reservoir with positive emotions. The higher the water level the more likely you are to be able to sail over the rocks of adversity rather than crash into them. Positive emotions buffer you against the storm, so that you're in a better position to survive the crisis. (*See* Chapter 8, Resilience.)

The positivity ratio – 3:1 positive to negative emotions

This is one of the most important discoveries to emerge from the science of well-being and, from my observations with clients, is the special ingredient that makes positive psychology coaching work. Here's the science bit …

When you experience more positive emotions than negative ones, at a ratio of 3 positive emotions to every 1 negative, you can enter into an upward spiral of growth. This spiral of development takes you into a place of greater well-being, which leads to positive change and flourishing. The upward spiral can even culminate in a personal transformation, the result of broadening your mind and opening you up to new knowledge, new skills, new people and new ways of being.[3]

That's three uplifting, positive emotional experiences to every one depressing, negative emotional experience. The ratio of 3:1 is the tipping point that divides a state of languishing (below 3:1) from a state of flourishing (above 3:1). Languishing is when you lack positive emotions and are neither fulfilling your potential nor realizing your goals. Flourishing, on the other hand, is when you feel positively toward life and you are succeeding in fulfilling your aspirations. People in depression typically operate at a positivity ratio below 1:1.[4]

This is a pearl of knowledge that holds the key to reversing the downward spiral into depression and initiating an upward spiral toward happiness and greater well-being. What it means is that for every negative emotional experience you suffer, you need an average of three positive emotional experiences to compensate, so that you can get on the track toward greater well-being above the tipping point of the positivity ratio.

I've seen the positivity ratio at work many a time with coaching clients. As they begin to feel better and their ratio increases, the more life begins to go well. You may recognize this from your own life – magical times when you were feeling good and everything you touched seemed to work out. We know that there is a relationship between happiness and success. Happiness is the result of success, but frequently experiencing positive emotions also seems to lead to success.[5] So, there's a virtuous cycle of happiness leading to success and vice versa.

I've also witnessed the positivity ratio leading to transformation in the work I've done with vulnerable young people that I mentioned earlier (*see* page 6). As they approached the positivity ratio, changes began to happen on the inside and outside. The transformation was visible in their physicality – they had more energy, clearer skin and a more groomed appearance. The transformation was internal but also external in the way their lives changed for the better, as they found jobs and better accommodation and got accepted on training courses.

Making the positivity ratio work for you

Here it is in a nutshell. The key to halting the downward spiral into depression is to aim for the positivity ratio, 3:1 in positive to negative emotions. So, how do you increase your experience of positive emotions? It helps to know something more about the nature of these delicate positive experiences.

Positive emotions generally arise as a result of the things we do and the way we see the world and interpret events in our lives. When you notice the good – what's right in your life rather than what's wrong – or do something that has a positive meaning for you, you'll be igniting a positive emotion. But you need to focus in to savour positivity and allow it to grow against the competition of 'louder' negative emotions.

'Don't fake it until you make it' with positive emotions. Feigning positivity to cover up negativity can lead to a toxic insincerity that stresses the body. You're aiming for a heartfelt positivity, grounded in reality, rather than something forced or fake or trivial. The rest of the book, in particular the next few chapters, has plenty of evidence-based techniques that will help you towards the positivity ratio. Think of it as your PE (Positive Emotions) Kit for well-being. Approach this with a lightness of touch, be open to the experience and remain relaxed about the outcome. Be patient – the effects are subtle and build over time. Here are a few practical things to consider, as you plan to climb the ladder of positive emotions.

✦ Ask yourself 'What's going right in my life right now? What is there to be pleased with? What is there to be grateful for?'

✦ Identify what you love doing and do more of it. What puts sunshine in your soul? What puts a spring in your step? Who do you love to be around?

✦ Engage wholeheartedly with a positive experience in the moment, without analyzing it. (This is the surest way of deflating your experience.)

✦ It's about the quantity more than the quality. Positive emotions are transient experiences, so accept their nature and let them pass. Instead, focus on increasing your quantity of positive emotional experiences.

✦ Keep the balance. It is possible to have too much positivity. The ratio breaks down at around 11:1 positive to negative emotions, so don't go overboard in your quest for more positive emotional experiences.

✦ Equally, you'll never get rid of negative emotions, which are entirely natural reactions, nor would it be desirable to eradicate them. Negative emotions have a function and provide the contrast, so that you can truly appreciate the positive when it happens.

Barbara Fredrickson recommends finding out what makes you come alive and giving those activities a higher priority. A lot of this is about prioritizing time to play, to love and to enjoy. In the time-crunched era we live in, where we're expected to be on call 24/7, time to play is increasingly rare in adult life. However, given the benefits of tapping into positive emotions, especially knowing that this is also a route to flourishing, isn't it worth dedicating some time to the things you truly love doing?

A playlist

In the same way that you might put together a playlist of your favourite tracks on an MP3 player, one idea to increase the frequency of your positive emotional experiences is to put together a list of things you enjoy doing and then commit to doing some of them on a regular basis. Recreational activities are ways to have fun, to explore something new and to put life's trials to one side. Try to do something at least once daily, if only for a quarter of an hour. Make sure it's something you can access easily. Active recreation, such as gardening or taking part in pub quizzes, is more satisfying and rewarding than passive leisure such as watching TV. Remember, it is the quantity of positive emotional experiences that counts. When I first did this, some of the things I had on my list included walks in the park, dancing *le roc* (French jive), meeting up with friends, going to perfume shops to smell all the lovely scents and visiting new cafés. Compile a list of some of your favourite activities and schedule something from your playlist to do every day.

PLAYLIST – THINGS I ENJOY ...

1. ....

....

2. ....

....

3. ....

....

→

4. ....

....

5. ....

....

6. ....

....

Based on Quality of Life Therapy[6]

Here's one final thought to inspire you to give yourself permission to enjoy life.

By investing in activities that generate positive emotions, you're investing in your future and opening yourself up to the possibility of a transformation.

The one to read: *Positivity* by Barbara Fredrickson

CHAPTER 4

Savouring the Moment

+ **What is it?** Savouring is the ability to tune into, appreciate and enhance the positive experiences in your life[1]

+ **In other words:** Extracting maximum enjoyment

+ **Try this for:** Enhancing the positive, happiness, positive emotions; building enjoyment of the present; as an aid to mindfulness, flow

+ **If you like this, try also:** Gratitude (Chapter 5) and Meditation (Chapter 6)

~

*It is a lovely sunny morning in August as I begin this chapter. I make my favourite breakfast – ripe, sweet, juicy berries of the season together with bloomy peaches and apricots. On top I add soya yogurt, which **tastes good*** as well as **doing me good**, and some healthy oats. I take breakfast into the garden, **luxuriating** in the warmth of the sun on my back and **feeling thankful** that I am able to start the working day this way. Every so often I take a break to harvest cherries, **marvelling** at how one small tree can produce so much fruit. I feel **grateful** to the previous owners, who planted this abundant tree. This year I've been baking with fresh cherries rather than preserving them as I usually do. Cherry pie and cherry and almond tart so far and **what's really good** is that it's eco-friendly as well as delicious with zero food miles! I'm **relishing** the idea next of making a cherry clafoutis, a French dessert that I last had when I lived in France during the 80s. One summer, I was helping out on a film shoot in Paris. Feeling shy I'd wander off at lunchtime, but one day the director sent someone to find me to join the crew in the bistro. They were missing me and wondering where I was. I felt **cherished** over lunch and **basked** in the warmth of their friendship. That was when I had the cherry clafoutis. Back in the garden I **appreciate** the blogger who has posted a recipe for cherry clafoutis online. Later I will be tucking into my first clafoutis in a quarter of a century. **Yum!**

~

In this short (but true) story are many of the features of savouring, processes that build positive emotions. Savouring is about appreciating the good. You'll be familiar with the usual meaning of savouring – to actively enjoy the taste of something. In positive psychology savouring is the capacity to appreciate and enhance positive experiences in life. It's about getting the full flavour of a positive experience, intensifying the enjoyment on offer. By *sharing* this story, I'm also using one of the strategies that maximize savouring.

Savouring can be applied to much more besides mouth-watering delicacies. Here's a random list to get you started:

✦ The beauty of nature – the landscape, the seasons, sunsets, rainbows.

✦ Time spent with loved ones, the warmth and support of friendships, the delight and innocence of young children, the wisdom of elders, the skills of colleagues, the kindness of strangers.

✦ A great book, a good film, a brilliant game, an uplifting concert, an inspiring piece of art or a fabulous piece of well-executed design.

✦ Simple pleasures such as a hug, a laugh, fresh bedlinen or a nice warm bath.

✦ Personal achievements, celebrations, special occasions such as birthdays, graduation, weddings, anniversaries.

You can savour almost anything. Savouring strengthens your awareness of the positive or the pleasurable to overcome the 'negativity bias'. Our brains are wired so that we notice what's wrong before we notice what's right, the negative before the positive. So if you're getting feedback on some task you've performed, you're more likely to hear the bad stuff than you are to take in the bits you did well in. You're more likely to notice the E you got in history than the As in science and geography. Savouring is a powerful tool to counter the negativity bias and it acts as a defence against negative emotions, helping you to bounce back from low moods.

Depression is almost a form of reverse savouring, where your awareness of the negative is intensified, 'savouring' the bleakness, the ashes and the utter grey-ness of life. This is what happened somewhat comically for a client of mine, when she headed to the local park for her first conscious attempt at savouring. Determined to savour all the lovely aromas of nature she breathed in deeply, but it was the smell of doggy doo-doo that assailed her senses!

When you get the hang of it, savouring is one of the principal positive psychology techniques, the key proc-ess in training your mind to notice what's good in life. It was by learning how to savour the positive that I was able to screen out more of the negative and begin the gradual process of recovery from depression. The five senses play a major role in the process of savouring.

✦ Some people favour the **visual** and will get a lot from feasting their eyes on something beautiful, such as a piece of art or a natural wonder.

✦ Others are more **auditory** and would relish the sound of great music, singing in a choir, birdsong or even the rainfall on a window when they're tucked up snug and warm indoors.

✦ Those who have **smell** as one of their stronger
senses have all the marvellous fragrances of nature
available to them, as well as the many scented
products. When I smell eau de cologne I am instantly
transported back to the many happy times spent
with my grandmother.

✦ Those who like **touch** will relish a hug or a massage
or a cuddle or a comforting warm bath.

✦ And of course there are the many wonderful **tastes**
of food. Some of my favourite flavours include the
spicy sweetness of satay, a creamy Brie, a ripe mango,
tart raspberries and the crisp elegance of a glass of
Sauvignon Blanc. I could go on! What works for you?

What do you enjoy savouring? Begin a list using the
senses as prompts – note your favourite sights, sounds,
fragrances and things to touch and taste. Below are some
ideas that you can add to for some sensory savouring.

~

*Savour the **sight** of … nature, dawn and sunset, the*
changing colours of the seasons, flowers, tall trees, pebbles
on the beach, a beautiful work of art, the many guises
of your favourite colour in both nature and products,
the kaleidoscope of colours in mosaics and stained glass,
houses with pastel-painted fronts

*Savour the **sound** of … music, your favourite radio show,*
the sea, rainfall, birdsong, bells, laughter, a language that
charms the ear

*Savour the **smell** of ... flowers, grass, perfumes and body lotions, suntan oil, scented candles, essential oils, baking, a barbecue*

*Savour the **feel** of ... walking barefoot on grass, a massage, a pet's fur, cool marble tiles, the sun on your skin, a furry hot water bottle*

*Savour the **taste** of ... your favourite foods*

And now – over to you ...

....

....

....

....

....

....

....

How to savour

Savouring is something that you do, a process rather than an end goal. Think of it as the journey rather than the destination. The more you cultivate savouring, the more you nurture positive emotions and increase your capacity to appreciate the good as it happens. Savouring requires your attention, although the more you practise it, the more likely it is to happen automatically. There are four key steps in savouring, with one caveat – relax and enjoy the process. Don't get hung up on whether you've got it right or not.

> • Slow down and stretch out the experience
> • Engage your full attention
> • Use all your senses
> • Reflect on the source of the enjoyment

The first step is a crucial one. Happiness and health generally increase as we slow down the pace of life. Slowing down, however, goes against the grain of the frantic pace of the 21st century with its fast tracking, instant messaging, fast food, etc, but it is vital to take your time when you want to maximize the enjoyment of a positive experience.

In workshops I bring out a bowl of exquisite fruit and chocolate truffles to savour. Eating a strawberry at half the speed and with twice the attention makes for an infinitely more pleasurable experience. Using the senses helps – notice a strawberry's bright red colour, its light fragrance, how the texture changes as you bite into it, and its sweet taste.

The *Slow Movement* is the very embodiment of savouring, a cultural shift towards slowing down the pace of life in order to fully appreciate its joys.[2] Best known of all is *Slow Food*, which is about taking the time to really appreciate the food you eat as well as the virtues of dining with friends, eating locally-sourced food with zero air miles (cherries from my tree for example) and slow cooking – think of how a casserole's flavour improves with time.[3]

The *Slow Movement's* many branches provide clues as to how we can apply savouring to various areas of life.

Slow Travel: Savouring the journey by engaging with local culture and people, rather than rushing to the destination and ticking off sights from your to-do list.

Slow Parenting: Letting kids have the time to be kids and enjoy their play rather than pressurizing them into early achievement at school or elsewhere.

Slow Cities: Making cities places that seek to improve the quality of life of their citizens with lots of green spaces and traffic-free zones for pedestrians.

Slow Sex: Slowing down to intensify the pleasure of physical intimacy. I'll leave the rest to your imagination!

The final step in savouring is about reflecting on the source of enjoyment. There is a subtle but important distinction here. It's about adding to the experience rather than analyzing it. So if you're savouring a strawberry you might be reflecting on thoughts of summer, strawberries and cream, tennis, etc; with a blueberry you might reflect on how it's a superfood, bursting with goodness.

To aid reflection a good question to ask is *'What's good about this?'* It works especially well if you're savouring something abstract, such as a memory. There is a tipping point though, where reflection spills over into analysis, so the best thing to do is to adopt an attitude of lightness and don't try too hard or think too much. I know exactly what this is like because of the terrible habit I used to have of asking the question 'But am I happy?' in the middle of an enjoyable experience. Net result – the happiness instantly deflated, punctured like a balloon. Engage with the experience rather than assessing it.

The risk of adversely affecting your enjoyment is shown by an experiment in which three groups were asked to listen to a recording of some classical music.[4] The first group simply listened to the music, the second were told to try to make themselves as happy as possible while listening to the music. The third group were asked to adjust a movable measurement scale to indicate their moment-by-moment level of happiness as they listened to the music. Which group do you think got the most enjoyment from savouring the music?

It was the first group who simply listened to the music, the second and third groups found their experience was compromised. When you focus too much on examining positive feelings, as opposed to just experiencing them, it may disrupt the pleasure and short-circuit the process of savouring.

Savouring processes

The leading researchers in the field are American psychologists Fred Bryant and Joseph Veroff, whose book *Savoring*[5] describes a number of strategies to encourage, prolong and intensify enjoyment of a positive experience.

Bryant and Veroff have boiled savouring down into four essential varieties: basking, luxuriating, marvelling and thanksgiving (gratitude). Gratitude is a powerful technique to increase happiness and reduce depression, which is why the next chapter is dedicated to it. Cherishing is another form of savouring within relationships (*see* Chapter 9).

These are all positive processes, but some have a shadow side. Too much basking transforms a sense of natural pride into arrogance. Luxuriating taken to excess could become overly self-indulgent. As with everything it is a case of balance. However, as depression puts you behind the starting line when it comes to savouring, give yourself permission to bask, luxuriate, etc, and let go of anxiety or moral judgment over the desirability of engaging in these processes.

Type of savouring	**BASKING**
What?	The warm enjoyment of a reflected accomplishment, when something that you have done is met with recognition, admiration or congratulations
Focus	Self
Experience	Reflection
Examples	Basking in praise, triumph, glory, the glow of a job well done
Results in	Pride (in its positive sense of recognizing your success)

Type of savouring	**LUXURIATING**
What?	Delighting in physical pleasures, enjoying bodily sensations
Focus	Self
Experience	Absorbed in something physical
Examples	Luxuriating in a nice warm bath, sun-bathing, sexual intimacy, a massage, a gourmet meal, fine wine, walking barefoot on grass, pampering, doing nothing
Results in	Physical pleasure

Type of Savouring	**MARVELLING**
What?	Transcending the self to experience a sense of wonder at something awe-inspiring or to commune with something bigger than the self
Focus	Outside the self
Experience	Absorbed in the sheer grandeur of something vast and/or impressive
Examples	Marvelling at nature, the Universe, the divine, a higher power, a person, science, technology, music, an achievement
Results in	Awe, wonder

Type of Savouring	**THANKSGIVING**
What?	Reflecting on your good fortune and being flooded with feelings of gratitude toward the agent of that positivity
Focus	Outside the self
Experience	Reflection
Examples	Becoming aware of a good thing in your life, winning against the odds, for example the lottery; near misses such as accidents, recovery from life-threatening illness
Results in	Gratitude

Based on Bryant and Veroff

Successful Savouring

There are some pre-requisites for savouring. First you have to be in a frame of mind where you are able to put aside concerns and worries, and secondly you need to be able to focus fully on the experience. Mindfulness techniques can help with both these aspects (*see* page 98) as can 'solo-tasking', the opposite of multi-tasking, where you focus attention on just one thing at a time. Developing a singular focus of attention can help with managing stress.

Savouring is, as the old saying goes, about slowing down to smell the roses. Having been a multi-tasking queen until I crashed into a mid-life depression, I now regularly stroll around my local park and stop to sample the fragrance of the roses, squeeze a stalk of lavender and appreciate the trees and their changing foliage. This break in the middle of a busy day has many benefits – it calms and it helps to clarify my thinking, so that I am in a better frame of mind to carry on with work. It's a win–win situation, as taking breaks to savour means I generally end up achieving more.

We know that savouring produces positive emotions and positive emotions broaden our thinking processes, enabling us to be more innovative and flexible thinkers. So here is a justification to take a break to slow down and savour!

One of the best ways of using savouring to lift your mood is to share the pleasure; this draws your attention to the array of delights on offer. Being in the company of others who are having a good time can help you be more open to enjoying yourself and they may point out some aspect of the pleasure that you've not yet clocked. Sharing a savouring experience helps to bond people and strengthens a relationship. It's not just participating either; the act of watching loved ones enjoying themselves is in itself pleasurable.

Sharing the experience is a particularly good approach for extroverts. If you are more introverted, you might prefer strategies that you can undertake alone, such as immersing yourself in what you're savouring. A way to encourage this is by consciously tuning in to certain stimuli (the beautiful, scented flowers growing by the roadside) while ignoring others (the cars). You can also take mental snapshots to build a memory of the source of pleasure. I did this on my first trip to Sydney, taking a ferry into the harbour with the Opera House on one side and the Harbour Bridge on the other. I immersed myself fully, drinking in every detail – marvelling at the feat of engineering that is the Harbour Bridge, appreciating the beauty of the shell-like curves of the Opera House and reflecting on its status as an icon of the Southern Hemisphere.

When something good happens, another way of cultivating savouring is to adopt expressive, exuberant behaviour, in which you speed up rather than slow down – whoop with joy, punch the air, bounce up and down, dance around. When you have performed well, give yourself a big pat on the back, reflect on how proud you are and think of how others will be impressed. It may feel counter-intuitive to give yourself such overt self-praise and can be inappropriate in certain situations, but there is evidence to suggest that outwardly expressing positive feelings can intensify them, so it is worth having a go.

Frequency of positive emotions has more of an impact on happiness than the intensity of them,[6] which means you're better off going for quantity rather than quality when it comes to savouring. Capitalize on the opportunities that come your way as you go about your day. A lot of savouring is reactive, such as marvelling at a rainbow after the rain, but here are also some ideas for pro-active savouring, beginning with a simple exercise.

DAILY SAVOURING

Once a day, take the time to slow down and enjoy something that you usually hurry through, for example eating a meal, walking somewhere or taking a shower. Afterwards write down what you did, how you did it differently and how it felt compared to when you usually rush through it.

Based on Positive Psychotherapy[7]

The savouring schedule

+ Plan your week with one formal, daily savouring session lasting at least 20 minutes.

+ Choose activities that you can look forward to and include variety in your schedule.

+ Everyday at the end of your session plan the next day's activity so you can relish the idea of it coming up. In the evening look back on that day's session to rekindle the good feelings involved.

+ At the end of the week, take some time to look back over all seven sessions and see if this re-ignites any of the positive feelings you had. Compare to how you would normally feel.

+ A similar idea is the Playlist (*see* page 52).

Based on Bryant and Veroff

PICTURE THIS!

This idea is something that has become much easier with the arrival of digital photography and smartphones with integrated cameras. Take a snapshot whenever you find yourself in an experience that you'd like to remember for future savouring. Make sure you stay engaged with the experience rather than thinking about camera angles etc. View the photos from time to time to savour the memories. You could post the pictures on a social media site to share the experience. Or embark on a mission to take one picture every day or on the first of each month to savour a whole year.

Modern technology acts as a great prop for savouring. I've found a smartphone to be invaluable for capturing the moment and creating a library of positive memories. I save the pictures as wallpaper for the phone and as screensavers on my computer. The images remind me of the joys of the moment, which I might otherwise forget. Research shows that the memories we recall tend to match the mood we're in, so the more negative the mood the more negative the memory. As depression leaves you with very little sense of the good times, digital snaps can provide you with a visual reminder of their existence.

Savouring across time

Savouring is often about appreciating the here and now, but you can also savour across time – bask in a happy memory or relish the anticipation of something pleasurable coming up.

Positive reminiscence

Positive reminiscence is about savouring pleasant memories from the past to boost happiness levels in the present, and is also used as a coping strategy to reduce emotional distress. The evidence suggests that people reminisce about past good times to gain insight and perspective to help them to manage current difficulties, feel better and escape from their problems. It works best when the positive reminiscing reminds you of your strengths, your abilities and good times, building confidence to deal with present difficulties. The risk comes when positive reminiscence is used solely as a means of escape, leading to negative comparisons with the present and living in the past.

Using a prompt or a prop can aid positive reminiscence. This might mean creating a picture in your mind linked to the memory, running through the events associated with it, sharing the story of it with someone, looking at memorabilia or playing music associated with that memory.

The senses play a role here, too, as the 19th-century French novelist Marcel Proust famously demonstrated in *Remembrance of Things Past*, in which memories are triggered by sensory experiences, such as sights, sounds and smells. The most famous instance is when the lead character eats a *madeleine*, a small tea cake, which transports him away from the dreariness and depression of the present to an experience of all-powerful joy.

Positive reminiscence can be especially beneficial for older people, for whom the past may provide a richer source of satisfaction than the present. It could, for example, be used as part of a 'life review' to generate a sense of personal achievement. Research shows that positive reminiscence can promote well-being and enhance self-esteem in older people. I interviewed many older people in my earlier work as a social historian and found that those who actively reminisced were among the happiest and liveliest of interviewees. This is confirmed by research on time orientation.[8] People who are heavily oriented towards a 'past positive' time perspective, which is associated with a warm, pleasurable view of their past, enjoy higher self-esteem and happiness.

Reminiscence can be a therapeutic process that brings together families, generations and communities. I've seen it used as a tool to facilitate friendships among older people who have shared memories of a particular time. Below is an activity to get you started on positive reminiscence.[9]

SAVOURING A HAPPY MEMORY

Compile a list of some of your happiest memories. It could be a golden period in your life, maybe your time at college, one of your best holidays, falling in love, the birth of a child, a work success, climbing a mountain, etc.

Next, pick one of those positive memories to reflect on. Relax, make sure you're sitting or lying down comfortably, take a deep breath, close your eyes and summon the memory to mind. Imagine the event in all its glory, allowing impressions to float freely across your consciousness. Run through the details. Notice who was present, the expressions on their faces, what was said, the environment you were in, the colours, the temperature, the ambience and the feelings you had at the time. Reflect on what was good about the experience.

This can be a co-coaching exercise, where one person savours a memory while the other one acts as the coach, encouraging reflection on the positive by asking, 'What was good about it?' Another variation, if you like writing, is to do it as a journaling activity where you write the story of the experience in rich, vivid detail.

Based on Bryant, Smart and King [9]

Savouring the future

Relishing the anticipation of something good that's coming up may seem out of reach in depression, however it offers benefits to those who succeed. Having something to look forward to creates hope, positive feelings about the future and motivation to ensure that the good thing is more likely to happen. Savouring something in the future gives you a chink of light in the darkness of depression. It is very easy to believe that there is nothing to look forward to, so this is where it helps to write a list of good things coming up, regardless of whether they excite you or not. This is about compiling evidence of good things existing in the future.

In periods of depression I write lists in my journal of things to look forward to. It could be something like getting together with a friend or summer being just around the corner. If you find there is absolutely nothing to look forward to, then that is your prompt to create something – schedule a get-together, a walk or an outing of some kind.

Allow yourself to fantasize about what is coming up. Visualization is a tool used a lot in positive psychology to set goals and develop optimism. Savouring something as yet unknown has both pros and cons. It can be a disadvantage in the sense that you may lack reference points to imagine how it will turn out, but it can also be an advantage in that you are therefore free to indulge in your fantasy without restriction. You can draw on the past as a reference point if you are repeating an activity. So, if you enjoyed the last time you went to stay with a friend, savour what was good about the experience and then project those same feelings forward to the next time you do it. Relish the anticipation.

There are two questions that help with savouring the future. Ask yourself:

✦ What is good about this?

✦ What am I looking forward to?

Many people find that the future is the most challenging of all the time dimensions to savour, regardless of whether they are experiencing depression. So stay relaxed about it and don't worry if it doesn't happen instantly.

Savouring is one of the foundations of positive psychology on which other techniques are built, hence it is worth mastering the art. By doing so you're opening yourself up to a wider and deeper experience of the pleasurable and positive.

The one to read: *Savoring* by Fred B. Bryant and Joseph Veroff

CHAPTER 5

The Attitude of Gratitude

✦ **What is it?** A feeling of thankfulness, wonder and appreciation for life

✦ **Try this for:** Happiness, positive emotions, satisfaction with life, relationships; as a cure for envy and disillusionment

✦ **If you like this, try also:** Savouring (Chapter 4) and Meditation (Chapter 6)

The author Sarah Ban Breathnach brought the 'gratitude journal' to international attention when she appeared on the Oprah Winfrey Show in the 90s and introduced a worldwide television audience to the idea of keeping a diary of the good things in life.[1] I was one of those watching and have kept a gratitude journal ever since. Many journal keepers describe it as life-changing; for me it has been the key to switching from a mindset of deprivation, aware of what was lacking in life, to one of abundance, appreciative of all the good things that I have. Gratitude improves your quality of life.

You may have grown up with a grandparent passing on the home-spun wisdom to 'count your blessings'. Well, it turns out that they were spot on. Gratitude has been proven by positive psychology research to be one of the most potent ways of increasing happiness and decreasing depression. Sonja Lyubomirsky, one of the leading researchers on happiness, describes gratitude as a 'meta-strategy' for achieving happiness, a superior level of technique.[2] This all comes from asking two simple questions: 'What is good in my life?' and 'What went well?'

The art of appreciation is about noticing what is right in your life rather than what is wrong, counting blessings rather than burdens. It is about training the mind to see where and how the glass is more full than empty. This helps to overcome the negativity bias, one of the barriers to happiness. Of course, when you're down it is a struggle to see any positives, but if you look hard enough you will find something to be thankful for, whether it is living in a safe area or that you are mobile and able to get from A to B. I tend to fall back on expressing gratitude for my home as the system that looks after my needs. So, I appreciate the pipes that bring in gas and water, the roof that keeps me dry, the walls that keep me warm, the electricity that powers the house, the phone and broadband that keep me connected, the computer that enables me to work from home, the garden that nourishes me, the view that inspires me, the neighbours who look out for me and I for them.

Robert Emmons, positive psychology's leading researcher on gratitude, describes it as a two-stage process, based on wanting what we have.[3] First, gratitude is about acknowledging what is good in your life. Secondly, it is about recognizing that the source of the good thing lies at least partially outside of yourself. Gratitude is, in essence, an appreciation of something external, an awareness of the benefits that we are not responsible for ourselves but are still fortunate to have. Developing the attitude of gratitude has a wide range of advantages for well-being. Research has shown that it's associated with increased happiness, satisfaction with life, self-esteem, positive emotions, optimism, hope, enthusiasm, empathy, vitality, spirituality and forgiveness. It's also linked to decreased depression, anxiety, loneliness, envy, neuroticism and materialism. What's not to love! Sonja Lyubomirsky identifies no fewer than eight ways in which the practice of gratitude builds happiness.[4]

✦ Encourages the savouring of positive life experiences

✦ Boosts self-esteem

✦ Helps you to cope with stress and adjust to difficult circumstances

✦ Deters negative emotions

✦ Promotes positive behaviour

✦ Nurtures relationships and reduces the likelihood of making unfavourable social comparisons to people you think are better off

✦ Mitigates against hedonic adaptation, where we take the good things in life for granted

✦ Leads to greater engagement with physical activity and fewer bodily ailments

Gratitude wears several hats in positive psychology. It is a positive emotion, so the more you experience it, the more you're opening yourself up to new possibilities, broadening your range of behaviour and building resources for your life. Practising gratitude will help you toward the positivity ratio and into a state of flourishing. It is also considered to be a strength, which is valued worldwide. Some people are stronger at feeling gratitude than others, but it is possible to develop your capability. Finally, gratitude is a strategy that increases happiness. The technique works best by stimulating positive emotions, so that we *feel* grateful rather than just thinking gratitude. This can be challenging when you're low and don't feel like doing a dry little exercise in your head. I certainly went a while before thinking gratitude in my head translated into a feeling of gratitude in my heart. But when it *does* work, gratitude becomes a powerful mood booster and a step toward the 'upward spiral' to greater emotional well-being. The key is to persevere while remaining relaxed about the outcome. Accept that sometimes it will connect to a positive emotion and sometimes it won't.

It is tricky to force yourself into feeling grateful, which is why Robert Emmons recommends trying instead to cultivate a *disposition* of gratefulness, which is the tendency to feel gratitude frequently.[5] People with a disposition to gratitude have a mindset that sees life as a gift. They notice the many blessings they receive. The clue is often in the language they use – grateful, thankful, blessed, gifts. Experiment with using the language of gratitude to turn it into a habit. It also helps to anchor gratitude to something you do as part of your routine, such as brushing your teeth or on your daily commute. I practise gratitude as part of a daily walk around the park. Noticing what's around me provides plenty of fuel for being thankful. Or, as psychologist David Pollay recommends, you could think of gratitude as having four foundation stones:[6]

+ First, gratitude reminds you of the **key people** in your life, who love and support you; this is significant because we know that having good relationships is a characteristic of happy people.

+ Secondly, gratitude acts as a reminder of your **strengths** – the natural talents that help you to move forward and reach goals.

+ Thirdly, gratitude for the things that you have already **achieved** reminds you of the road already travelled.

+ Finally, gratitude acts as a reminder of the **wonders of the world** such as the miracles of nature, which show how mighty oaks can grow from tiny acorns. That growth can occur from the smallest of beginnings is an optimistic thought.

Gratitude is a positive emotion often associated with the past (appreciating what has been gained), but it can also help to generate positive emotions about the future. Having the evidence of things that went well before promotes a confidence in the possibility of things going well in the future, too. Gratitude is the glass half full looking back, whereas optimism is the glass half full looking forward. Gratitude can stimulate optimism, which makes it doubly valuable as optimism (*see* Chapter 7) is one of the key strategies that promote happiness.

A cynic would say that it is all very well feeling thankful when things are working out in your life, but what about when you have suffered a misfortune and are feeling down? Gratitude sometimes requires a degree of contrast or deprivation in order to experience its full effects as a positive emotion according to Robert Emmons. So while no one would ever recommend a loss of some kind, it does mean that when a need is filled after a period of absence, you will have a sweeter experience of gratitude. You appreciate the rain after months of drought or new work after a job loss.

Losing something of value in one area of life can lead to a greater appreciation in other areas. The stressed-out executive, who quits his job to 'spend more time with the family', may experience a fresh appreciation of his children, which might not have been the case had he continued his high-pressure lifestyle.

Stressful events can act as a prompt for gratitude. I remember feeling flooded with heart-felt appreciation the first time I had surgery. Being confronted with the reality of mortality renews appreciation for life itself; there was gratitude for the friends who supported me through the surgery and appreciation for the care given by the medical staff who restored me back to health. Imagining the bad stuff that might have happened but didn't, can spark a torrent of appreciation – a near miss in the car, getting the 'all-clear' diagnosis or keeping your job during a wave of redundancies. Research indicates that people who engage in this positive counterfactual thinking tend to be happier than those who don't.[7] There is also evidence to suggest that those who are able to be grateful in the wake of a trauma, such as being thankful that you still have something like your health or sanity, are better equipped to cope positively with the distress. They may even experience personal growth as a result of finding some benefit or silver lining in the trauma, such as a renewed appreciation for life (*see* Post-Traumatic Growth, page 159).

Gratitude is an antidote to rumination, the enemy of well-being and a feature of depression in which the mind obsesses endlessly over negative events and personal failings.[8] Some psychologists recommend practising gratitude as a cure for envy, which has a lack of appreciation for what you *do* have at its core. It has also been suggested as an antidote for excessive materialism with all that goes with it, such as resentment, disappointment and bitterness. This is something that you can extend to your professional life as well as the personal. So, for example, if you are dissatisfied with your job and feel disillusioned, then one idea is to make a note of all the positives that your work brings you, money being one of the most obvious! This can help to protect you from the trap of disengagement and acts of self-sabotage at work.

Gratitude techniques: three good things

Cultivating the art of appreciation doesn't require material wealth but rather an attitude of thankfulness regardless of current circumstances. One of the simplest and most powerful ways of practising gratitude is through an exercise called 'three good things' or 'three blessings'. The way to do it is to think of three specific things that are good in your life or have gone well for you. You can do this at bedtime as a means of reflecting on the day – it leads to improved sleep and a greater sense of refreshment on waking up. But it can be done at any point in the day, for example at mealtimes or on your commute. This technique was included in Martin Seligman's early experiments with positive psychology interventions and was shown to lead to a lasting increase in happiness and decrease in depression with the effects felt months later.[9]

Something that is good in your life could be a big thing, such as having a place to call your own, or it could be something personal, such as a positive relationship with someone. The good thing could also be something small like getting the last seat on the bus. Something that has gone well could be a big achievement, such as passing a test, or a smaller one like managing to get the recycling done. In depression motivation is very limited, so it is especially important to appreciate the smallest of achievements. Follow the advice to do just one small thing a day. So, if you manage to get yourself to the park, regardless of how far you walk, then that is something to include as one of your three good things. Celebrate the progress no matter how small. If you manage to do a complete circuit of the park whereas before you only managed half a circuit, then that is something to include on your list. Once you get into the habit of gratitude, you often spot things during the day that will make it onto the gratitude list later.

Here are some ideas to get you started (make these personal and specific to you).

GRATITUDE LIST

✔ Health

✔ Home

✔ Neighbourhood

✔ Family

✔ Friends

✔ Pets

✔ People who support you

✔ Organizations that have helped you

✔ Work

✔ Living in a safe country

✔ Nature

✔ A temperate climate

You can add to the benefits of gratitude by looking at what your involvement might have been in making the good things happen. This builds confidence as you notice the link between your actions and the good things it results in later. Say months ago you came across some work project that sparked your curiosity. It could be your action in registering an interest in the project that influences you landing work on it months later. Life rewards action.

The challenge can be to find new ways of showing gratitude to keep the practice varied and fresh. For that David Pollay suggests 'gratitude chains'. Take the baked beans on your plate. Someone will have grown those beans, harvested them, packed them, shipped them, stocked them and then sold them to you. So there's a chain of gratitude to all the people who played their role in getting the food to your table. The beans were kept in your kitchen cupboard, which presents another opportunity for a 'gratitude chain'; gratitude to nature for growing the tree that became the wood that went into the cupboard; gratitude to the carpenter who made the cupboard and to the people who transported it to your home. You can also appreciate the qualities of the objects themselves. So, in this example you might appreciate the wood for its strength (and reliability) in keeping your food safe and off the floor.

'Three good things' can be used as a coaching or therapy technique to focus a client's attention on what is working well in their life. I use it at the start of a session to help the client into a positive, resourceful frame of mind. It is also a good bedtime routine to get into with young children to nurture the development of a grateful disposition in them. By encouraging children to reflect on the good things in their lives, you are helping them to develop a mindset of appreciation rather than an awareness of what's missing.

Gratitude is also a great technique to teach to young people. When I do group work I begin by getting the participants to check in with 'three good things' as a way of keeping track on what has gone well and progress made since the previous session. In the study I ran with vulnerable young people misusing alcohol, gratitude came out as the most successful of all the strategies used to raise happiness and the one that was still practised after the end of the programme. This not only holds true for adolescents living on the margins of society, but also for the most privileged young people. Wellington College, one of the UK's best-known independent schools, has run a well-being programme for a number of years, an initiative of the headmaster Anthony Seldon. I asked one of the teachers which of all the well-being interventions had had the most impact on the students. Gratitude ranked alongside meditation in top position.

The gratitude journal

The idea behind the gratitude journal is to record a list of the good things in your life. This is an extended version of 'three good things', a 'good news journal', which is the antithesis of the doleful Dear Diary, in which many of us recorded our deepest fears as angst-ridden teenagers. The act of writing it in a journal helps to process your thoughts and raise awareness of the good that *does* exist in your life, as well as your role in making it happen. Each time aim to record at least five things that have gone well or are having a positive effect on your life. As with 'three good things' these can be big or small, temporary or on-going. This is something that can be done daily, however research favours doing it less frequently, such as once a week, which prevents it from becoming a chore. I do it on a Sunday evening, which is a good moment to reflect back on the week that's been and also to look ahead. Choose a notebook that you will treasure (the savouring begins here) and a pen in your favourite shade of ink. You can also get gratitude apps for smartphones if you prefer a high-tech version.

- *What is good in my life today?*
- *What went well today?*
- *What part did I play in making the good thing happen?*

The gratitude journal is a mighty tool in developing a mindset of abundance. As we look back over our lives it is all too easy to recall losses, missed opportunities, rela-tionship breakdowns and the plethora of pain that we accumulate as we get older. The gratitude journal con-tains the evidence of all the good times and things in your life, which you may easily forget. As I look back over my old journals, it is like getting another taste of the good times and another opportunity to savour the good in life.

Less is more. The gratitude journal works best when you do it less frequently, say, once a week rather than daily.

Thank-you therapy

A great way of amplifying the benefits of practising gratitude is to express it to others, thanking people for things they have done for you. Gratitude nurtures relationships, helping them to flourish. It is enriching for both the giver and receiver, setting up a loop of happiness in which your gratitude makes both you and the recipient feel good and the goodwill then bounces back and forth between you. A friend of mine, Clive, did his own experiment with gratitude while we were training in positive psychology. He wrote handwritten notes using quality paper and envelopes to express thanks for good service he had received – for example, taking the time to thank the owners of a go-kart business who'd laid on a birthday treat to which his son was invited and to thank the owners of a deli that had recently opened. On both occasions Clive was specific in his thanks and each time he received a note back thanking him for his thanks! Gratitude is a great way of connecting with people, and connections such as these can bring richness into life. This shows how gratitude can act as a social lubricant, facilitating relationships in your community. It also stops you taking people for granted. We often value our relationships during a moment of crisis, but expressing gratitude to someone enables us to appreciate those special people as part of the everyday rather than in exceptional circumstances. In one of the first studies of positive psychology interventions, participants were asked to write a letter of thanks to someone who was a positive influence on them in the past, such as a teacher or a relative. They then delivered the letter in person reading it out loud to them in a 'gratitude visit'. The results were an immediate and substantial boost to happiness, although the effects weren't as enduring as with 'three good things'.[10]

A NOTE OF THANKS

Dear................,

I'm writing to thank you for the support you have given me in the past when ....

....

Writing a thank-you note is an act of thanksgiving and a form of savouring (see page 54) with a doubly uplifting effect for you and the recipient. Writing a card also creates an event to savour. Use stationery that is visually appealing or has a luxurious texture, play music that puts you into a good mood and treat yourself to something delicious as you write your note of thanks. If you want to upscale the art

→

of appreciation, you could host a gratitude party for everyone you'd like to thank. The research indicates that you get better results from performing acts of kindness in a short time-span, so try expressing your thanks in one day or event to maximize the positive emotions.

Appreciative Inquiry

The art of appreciation is making its way into the workplace in the form of 'Appreciative Inquiry' or AI, a process of organizational development which is centred on the belief that every person or group has something good to offer. The first step in AI is to appreciate the existing skills and talents across the staff, asking questions such as 'What's working?' and 'What's good about what you're currently doing?'[11] The process of change is then based on the assets of an organization rather than its deficiencies. You can use a similar approach to other groups in your life to stimulate thankfulness: what's good about your family, friends, colleagues, neighbourhood or community? What's working well? What is there to appreciate?

The one to read: *Thanks! How the New Science of Gratitude Can Make You Happier* by Robert Emmons

CHAPTER 6

Meditation: The Mindful Approach

✦ **What is it?** Meditation is a practice that calms the mind and relaxes the body

✦ **Mindfulness** is about paying attention in a non-judgmental way[1]

✦ **In other words:** Being present, letting go, detaching from negative thoughts and feelings, a human 'being' rather than a human 'doing'

✦ **Try this for:** Reducing depression and anxiety; positive emotions, relaxation

✦ **If you like this, try also:** Savouring (Chapter 4) and Vitality (Chapter 10)

They say that laughter is the best medicine and if you're in a sprint for a quick mood boost then that will certainly work. However, if you're in the marathon for a sustainable mood improvement, then meditation would surely be up among the medal-winners. I first became convinced of the merits of meditation for depression when I discovered an experiment from neuroscience that showed that regular practice of mindfulness meditation activates the part of the brain associated with positive emotions – the left prefrontal cortex.[2] Yes, it seems that meditation can *grow* your capacity to experience happiness.

Lean to the left

Dr Richard Davidson is the neuroscientist who has examined the effects of meditation on the brain. His research indicates a left-right division in the brain's set points for mood. When people are emotionally distressed – anxious, depressed and angry – the most active sites in the brain are around the amygdalae (centres of fear) and the right prefrontal cortex. When people are in a good mood, those sites are quiet with heightened activity instead in the left prefrontal cortex. Davidson discovered that a quick way of working out a person's typical mood range is to assess the activity in these left and right prefrontal areas. The more the activity tilts to the right, the more unhappy a person tends to be, while the more activity there is on the left, the more happy they are. Davidson has taken readings from hundreds of people, including Buddhist monks, and found that regular meditators have much higher activation on the left-hand side.[3]

To anyone in depression it is like sweet music to the ears to hear that meditation is a means to develop that 'muscle' for joy, love, contentment and other positive emotions. I was inspired to try the experiment for myself, practising mindfulness meditation daily over eight weeks and yes, it did work. I experienced more positive emotions, though I might not have recognized them if I hadn't been keeping a mood diary as this was a 'quieter' experience of positive emotions rather than the high notes of bliss and ecstasy. Instead, I felt calm, relaxed and less anxious. It was a joyful relief after many years of stress and marked a turning point in my life. I went from believing that I might be incapable of happiness to realizing that I was, in fact, consumed by stress. Through meditation I calmed down a perpetually busy mind and was more able to tune into life's joys. My ability to savour increased, too. I was at a friend's home one evening when her cat came in from outdoors. I leaned over to stroke Louis and found myself going into raptures over his 'chilled fur'!

Meditation has been a part of spiritual practice for thousands of years in Eastern religions, most notably in Buddhism. There are two broad styles in meditation – concentration and mindfulness, which are frequently combined. Concentration involves focusing attention in a sustained fashion on one object and, when the attention wanders, bringing it back to that one thing. It could be a candle flame, your breath or a mantra that you repeat over and over. In concentration meditations, you continually return your attention to a central focus.

Mindfulness is somewhat different. There is no particular focus involved, it is instead a process of paying attention to your ongoing experience, whatever it may be at that moment. So, if you have lower back pain and that happens to be prominent in your awareness right now, you pay attention to that – not by trying to concentrate on it, but simply by noticing it and letting it be. You don't try to make it different or hold onto it. You just notice it as fully as you can, including what is going through your mind about it. It's about observation rather than reaction, monitoring rather than reacting to the content of your experiences.

With practice this is a way of gaining awareness of the nature of our emotional and thought patterns, which enables us to step back and stop reacting in a knee-jerk fashion to stress triggers. When adversity strikes many of us respond as though we're on autopilot. We interpret stressful events as uncontrollable and threatening. Meditation training, however, allows us some distance, so we have more of a bird's eye view on a situation and therefore more flexibility in the way we respond to the trigger.[4] Flexibility of thinking is one of the key tools of resilience, the ability to bounce back from adversity (see Chapter 8).

Meditation began as a spiritual ritual in the East and has now been adopted as a health practice in the West. There has been extensive research on the benefits of practising meditation for your psychological well-being. The big question here is which form of meditation works best to increase happiness and reduce depression? Both loving-kindness and mindfulness meditations have come under the scrutiny of psychologists, loving-kindness for its power to increase positive emotions and mindfulness for its ability to reduce depression and anxiety.

BENEFITS OF MEDITATION

MORE	LESS
✔ Positive emotions	✘ Depression
✔ Happiness	✘ Stress
✔ Resilience	✘ Anxiety
✔ Ability to handle stress	✘ Loneliness
✔ Ability to relax	✘ Hostility
✔ Satisfaction with life	✘ Neuroticism
✔ Energy	✘ Pain
✔ Openness	✘ Relationship issues
✔ Self-esteem	✘ Negative body image
✔ Self-acceptance	
✔ Self-actualization	
✔ Creativity	
✔ Enthusiasm	
✔ Learning ability	
✔ Trust	
✔ Self-control	
✔ Empathy	
✔ Spirituality	

Loving-kindness meditation

This is one of Buddhism's most ancient meditations and involves cultivating positive emotional states of love and kindness toward ourselves and others, so that we become more patient, accepting and compassionate. According to Buddhist theory happiness comes through empathizing with others and seeing their suffering and well-being as equally important as our own. By recognizing that one of our needs is to help others meet their needs, we shed a layer of self-centredness and find a path toward happiness.

Barbara Fredrickson, the scientist renowned for her work on positivity, was curious to know what effect loving-kindness meditation might have on our emotions. She ran an experiment asking individuals to focus daily on their hearts and to direct loving, kind feelings toward themselves, then to loved ones, acquaintances, strangers, and finally, all sentient beings.[5] The results of the experiment showed that practising loving-kindness meditation increases a wide range of positive emotions, including love, joy, gratitude, contentment, hope, pride, amusement and awe. The rise in positive emotions was matched by a decline in symptoms of depression and an improved sense of satisfaction with life. Other benefits included an increase in self-acceptance, positive relationships and good physical health.

Loving-kindness meditation could be used as a way to reach for that optimal 3:1 positivity ratio that I mentioned earlier (*see* page 47), where people begin to flourish when they average three or more positive emotions for every one negative emotion. Barbara Fredrickson also recommends loving-kindness meditation as a remedy for one of the biggest challenges in positive psychology – the 'hedonic treadmill'. This is where we start to take for granted the sources of our happiness, so that they have less of an effect on us. The third time you go back to that prize-winning restaurant is never as good as the first time. We even become accustomed to the ultimate joy of falling in love. Loving-kindness meditation produces such a wide range of increased positive emotions in a broad variety of situations that it helps to keep things fresh and to outpace this 'hedonic treadmill'.

THE 'HOW TO' OF LOVING-KINDNESS MEDITATION (METTA BHAVANA)

Loving-kindness is the first in a series of meditations in Buddhism that produce four qualities of love, starting with friendliness (*metta*), then compassion (*karuna*), appreciative joy (*mudita*) and equanimity (*upekkha*). You might want to get hold of a guided meditation or try your nearest Buddhist centre to learn how to develop the practice.[6] Approach this meditation with an open heart toward yourself and others.

- Begin with directing a loving acceptance toward yourself. You may experience resistance initially to the idea of this but the practice of this meditation is designed to overcome self-doubt and negativity.

- Send loving-kindness toward yourself and then systematically to each of these four types of people:

  1. Someone you respect such as a spiritual teacher
  2. Someone you love dearly and unconditionally – a close family member or a friend
  3. A neutral person – somebody you know, but have no special feelings toward, such as an acquaintance or someone who serves you in a shop
  4. A hostile person – someone you are currently having difficulty with

The intention behind loving-kindness meditation is to break down the barriers between you and these four types of people with a parallel effect of also breaking down divisions within your own mind, the source of much of the conflict we experience. Try using different people to whom you send loving-kindness, as some won't fit easily into the categories above, but keep to the prescribed order. Here are some hints to help develop feelings of loving-kindness. Keep your focus on the positive feelings your practice arouses, rather than on the technique itself:

✦ **Visualization** – bring to mind a picture of the person the feeling is directed at and imagine them smiling at you or simply being joyous.

✦ **Reflection** – reflect on the positive qualities of the person and their acts of kindness. Reflect, too, on your own positive qualities and make positive affirmations about yourself.

✦ **Auditory** – repeat a mantra or a phrase to yourself such as 'loving-kindness'.

Loving-kindness is a meditation of the heart. Buddhists suggest that it should be seen as more than a formal sitting practice removed from everyday life. They recommend taking it out into the world and directing a friendly attitude and openness toward everyone you relate to.

Mindfulness meditation

'Mindfulness' means 'awareness' or 'bare attention'. It is about being fully awake to the here and now, living in the present, connected to the flow of every experience and conscious of the body–mind connection. Mindfulness in practice is a way of paying attention to the present moment, so that we become more aware of our thoughts and feelings and as a consequence are more able to manage them rather than be overwhelmed by them. The opposite is mindlessness, a feeling of being on auto-pilot, disconnected, obsessed with the past or fearing the future. Mind*less*ness is a way of wandering through life reacting automatically to people and situations, succumbing to habits such as stuffing yourself with food without noticing what you're eating or wasting endless hours in front of the TV. Mindless habits like these often steer us off-course on the road to happiness and well-being.

Psychologists have found there to be a number of benefits from practising mindfulness, which is why it is being adopted as a health practice, known for its ability to soothe the mind.

MINDFULNESS ...[7]

- Helps us to experience the world directly without the endless commentary of our thoughts.

- Helps us to experience thoughts as mental events that come and go like clouds and as ideas that aren't necessarily true.

- Helps us to live in the present rather than dwelling on the past or worrying about the future.

- Helps us to become more self-aware and stops us coasting on 'autopilot'.

- Helps to interrupt the cycle of mental events that cause us to spiral into depression.

- Stops us from trying to force life to be a certain way and helps us to become more accepting of what is.

People who practise mindfulness are less likely to experience distress – they have a greater understanding and acceptance of their emotions and recover from bad moods faster. They also have less frequent negative thoughts and are more able to let them go when they arise. Mindful people feel more in control and have a greater ability to override or change their internal thoughts and feelings, so that they avoid acting on impulse. They have higher, more stable self-esteem that is less dependent on external factors.

Mindfulness meditation is now recognized as a treatment for depression and as a prevention strategy to stop people relapsing into depression. It is particularly helpful in dealing with the effects of stress and can reverse the symptoms of the chronic stress response. Stress strengthens the negative networks in the brain and weakens positive ones. It prevents the creation of new neural connections, which can in turn lead to burnout. By staying in the present you avoid being overly oriented to past stresses, which can trigger depression, or overly oriented toward future stresses, which can set off anxiety. Mindfulness helps you to respond to stressful situations in a more reflective style, rather than reacting automatically to try and deflect the pain.

The Buddhist monk Thích Nhât Hạnh describes this as avoiding the urge to chase away unpleasant feelings and choosing the more effective path of observing the feeling quietly, giving it a name such as sorrow or anger and returning to your breathing. This helps us to recognize and identify the feeling more clearly.[8] Rather than engaging with the negative feeling or thought and trying to suppress it, mindfulness encourages us to observe and be more accepting of it. Attempting to avoid or alter the intensity or frequency of an unwanted mental experience can – paradoxically – keep it going and set off all the familiar triggers. By accepting rather than resisting unpleasant feelings, we may find that they go away by themselves. What you resist persists. Equally, when we give up trying to force pleasant feelings, they are freer to emerge on their own. Experienced meditators suggest that when we stop trying to make something happen, a whole world of fresh and unanticipated experiences can open up.

My own practice tells me the truth of this. By taking regular breaks to meditate and letting go of always being in control, I found that there was rarely a cost but plenty of good, unexpected things occurred, which seemed to be more than coincidence. The most memorable was the day when my meditation was interrupted late on by a phone call from a media company. They were interested in using my house as a location for filming a viral marketing campaign. This was most welcome as I had returned to studying and was keen on finding alternative ways of covering my bills. Later that day they came and took some test shots and my kitchen was selected as a location. A week later they were in, filming a satire on the celebrity chef Gordon Ramsay. 'Little Gordon' rapidly became an Internet sensation, gathering several million hits online with my kitchen gaining worldwide exposure, even making it onto primetime American TV. So, as I developed my meditation practice the changes that occurred weren't just on the inside; life began to change on the outside, too.

Evidence from neuroscience has confirmed the many benefits of mindfulness meditation, including its effectiveness in reducing anxiety and negative emotions.[9] People who undergo mindfulness training show the increase in activation of the left prefrontal cortex, the area of the brain associated with positive emotions, which is generally less active in people who are depressed. What this means, in effect, is that the more you meditate the more you develop your capacity for positive emotions and happiness. The best-known therapeutic programmes are Mindfulness-Based Stress Reduction (MBSR) and Mindfulness-Based Cognitive Therapy (MBCT). Other programmes such as Acceptance and Commitment Therapy (ACT) and Dialectical Behaviour Therapy (DBT) also contain elements of mindfulness.

Mindfulness-Based Stress Reduction (MBSR)

One of the leading practitioners of the mindful approach to health is Jon Kabat-Zinn, who developed Mindfulness-Based Stress Reduction (MBSR)[10] at the University of Massachusetts Medical Center in the late 1970s. MBSR has been used with tens of thousands of hospital patients with a variety of psychological and physical illnesses, such as generalized anxiety disorder, chronic pain, cancer, fibromyalgia and multiple sclerosis, and has a track record of reducing anxiety and depression.[11] MBSR training is general rather than tailored to any particular diagnosis and has now extended beyond clinical settings into the wider community.

Mindfulness-Based Cognitive Therapy (MBCT)

Mindfulness-Based Cognitive Therapy (MBCT)[12] brings together MBSR with Cognitive-Behavioural Therapy (CBT). Mindfulness differs from CBT in that it doesn't encourage people to challenge their thoughts but rather to accept those thoughts without identifying with them. People are told not to aim for a particular result, but simply to practise mindfulness and see what happens. MBCT was developed in the 1990s to train people who suffer recurrent depressive episodes in techniques that disengage from automatic negative thinking, which can precipitate depression in susceptible individuals. Rumination, in which the mind repeatedly reruns negative thoughts, is a key factor in people relapsing into depression, and even minor increases in sadness can reactivate the neural pathways of depressive thinking. Mindfulness is an alternative way of experiencing negative emotions that can prevent those emotions leading to depression. MBCT teaches people how to shift mental gears to avoid being dragged into the downward spiral. The experts behind MBSR and MBCT have collaborated on *The Mindful Way through Depression*[13] with a CD of meditations narrated by Jon Kabat-Zinn.

> ### FIRST STEPS TO MINDFULNESS
>
> 1. Whenever possible just do one thing at a time.
>
> 2. Pay full attention to what it is that you are doing.
>
> 3. When your mind wanders from this, gently bring it back.

Kabat-Zinn suggests that bringing even a tiny bit of awareness to a single moment can help to break the chain of events that leads to chronic unhappiness. Start by choosing some routine activity that you do everyday and resolve to do it mindfully bringing a moment-by-moment awareness to the task. Applying mindfulness to the washing up is a classic way of developing the practice. So you might notice the sensations as you put your hands into the warm water in the sink, how the temperature changes as you adjust the hot and cold taps, the aroma of the washing-up liquid, the rhythm of washing and stacking plates, the twinkling of newly-washed cutlery, the contrast as the crockery goes from dirty to clean and the feeling of completion when the task is done. You can also apply this mindful approach to other domestic tasks as well as to eating, brushing teeth, showering or driving. Directly sensing the messages that the body is giving us reduces the persistent mental chatter going on in our heads.

Mindfulness practices

Mindfulness has been around for thousands of years. Below are some simple steps to get you started on some of the practices. You could also join one of the mindfulness programmes like MBSR or MBCT, which typically run for eight weeks. A brief web search will reveal the nearest location to you.

MINDFUL BREATHING

1. Find a comfortable position either sitting or lying down. If you are sitting down, make sure your back is straight and allow your shoulders to drop.

2. Close your eyes.

3. Focus your attention on your breathing. Notice what it feels like in your body to slowly breathe in and out. Make sure you are breathing correctly – that as you breathe in, your belly expands.

4. Now pay attention to your belly; feel it rise and expand every time you breathe in and feel it sink as you breathe out.

5. Immerse yourself fully in the complete experience of your breathing.

6. Whenever you notice your mind wandering away from your breath, simply notice what it was that

→

took your attention away and then return to your breathing in the present moment.

7. Continue for 10 minutes or more if you prefer.

MINDFULNESS ON THE MOVE

Some people prefer a more active form of meditation to the sitting practice of mindful breathing, where we withdraw our attention from the outside world. Walking mindfully is a form of meditation on the move with a greater awareness of what's going on on the outside – the environment, the elements, the people – while maintaining a focus on the experience of walking. It is a good way of increasing awareness of our physical bodies. For your first attempt find an open space, such as a park, where you can walk uninterrupted for 15 to 20 minutes without having to deal with any traffic.

1. As you stand on the spot, notice how your weight connects to the earth through your feet. Note the sensation of your feet in contact with the ground, your shoes, socks etc. Let your arms hang naturally as you begin to walk.

2. Walk normally, but slow down the pace to increase awareness. Keep your attention on

→

the soles of your feet. Note how you lift and drop your foot, the contact with the ground, followed by the release and how your body shifts with each step.

3. Take your attention up through your body as you walk allowing each part to relax.

4. Notice what emotions happen to be present and what is going on in your mind. When thoughts unrelated to walking come up, just let them fade and return your attention to the experience of moving.

5. Keep a balance between your awareness of the outer and inner worlds.

Once you've got the hang of this, every routine journey becomes an opportunity for mindfulness on the move.

THE RAISIN EXERCISE

This is an exercise that many therapists use to introduce their clients to the detail involved in attending to something mindfully. You don't have to use raisins, but choose a food that is small and easy to handle, such as grapes or blueberries.

→

1. Spend a minute looking at the raisin, noticing its colour and texture. Then take a moment to notice its scent.

2. Next, put the raisin in your mouth but don't chew it. Move it around your mouth and feel its texture with your tongue.

3. Then, take one small bite out of the raisin. Notice the difference between the taste and the texture of the skin and flesh of the fruit.

4. Once you've noticed everything there is to notice, try eating the raisin slowly, aware of everything you taste and feel.

You may have noticed that mindfulness has a lot in common with savouring. Indeed, it does but they are cousins rather than twins. Emotions may or may not be involved in mindfulness, but they are the target of savouring.

THE BODY SCAN MEDITATION

This is a mindfulness exercise that helps us get a sense in the moment of what's going on in our internal landscape with our physical and emotional sensations. The body scan is a good way to ground

→

or centre yourself and can also be used as such after an upsetting situation. I recommend lying down and taking your time to check in with each body part slowly and in detail, but you can also do it standing up. Get hold of a guided meditation to talk you through the exercise or, alternatively, put on some relaxing music to accompany your meditation.

1. Lie down, make sure you are comfortable, close your eyes and begin by getting in touch with your breathing. Notice where your body makes contact with the bed or the floor. Take a few deep breaths to ground yourself.

2. Start either with the toes of one foot or the crown of the head and slowly scan your attention up or down depending on your starting point. The idea is simply to feel deeply into each part – whether bone, muscle, organs or blood flow, and notice what is present in your body. Note what is tense, relaxed, hot, cold, numb, tingling. Whatever is present in your body in that moment is what you pay attention to.

3. Adopt an attitude of gentle curiosity to investigate the quality of the sensations that you find. The intention is simply to notice what is, not to feel different or to relax, although this may be a happy consequence.

4. Move along in sequence, so if you start with the toes of one leg, move slowly upward. Notice what is happening in your feet, calves, knees, thighs, pelvic region, lower back, stomach, mid-back, chest, shoulders, arms, hands, neck, face and head. Spend a few minutes in each area deepening your awareness into whatever is present.

5. When the mind wanders, acknowledge it noticing the thoughts and emotions, remain mindful and gently return your attention to your breath and the part you were scanning.

6. Don't worry about getting it right or whether it is 'working' or not. The scan is a way of reconnecting on a deeper level with your body and recognizing the links between bodily sensations, thoughts and emotions.

The one to read: *The Mindful Way Through Depression* by Mark Williams, John Teasdale, Zindel Segal and Jon Kabat-Zinn

The Mental Health Foundation has a website devoted to mindfulness – www.bemindful.co.uk

CHAPTER 7

Learning Optimism: Psychological Self-defence

✦ **What is it?** Expecting a positive outcome, a sense of confidence about things turning out well

✦ **In other words:** The glass is half full

✦ **Try this for:** Overcoming pessimism and negative thinking

✦ **If you like this, try also:** Positive Emotions (Chapter 3) and Resilience (Chapter 8)

I was convinced for many years that I was a natural-born pessimist but, even if I wasn't born a pessimist, circumstances had certainly contrived to turn me into one. I expected that life would be hard and believed that the only way to succeed was to put in masses of work and make multiple sacrifices to overcome the odds. Not surprisingly, I was prone to episodes of depression. The turning point came one winter when I was on my way home from a ski trip in the Alps. It was snowing hard by the time I reached Geneva airport and all flights had been grounded. My mood turned as bleak as the sky. I was stuck at the airport just like I was stuck in life. Nothing was ever going to change. I slumped into a seat, resigned to a long wait and reached into my luggage for something to read. I fished out *Learned Optimism* by Martin Seligman and found out that it was possible to develop optimism even if you were born a pessimist. Pessimism isn't fixed. This was the revelation that gave me the confidence that life could change and ultimately put me on track for greater happiness.

Both optimism and pessimism influence the way we think and feel when we encounter problems. Optimists expect good outcomes even in difficult situations, which leads to a relatively positive mix of feelings, whereas pessimists expect bad outcomes and this yields more negative feelings, such as anxiety, anger, sadness and despair.[1] One of the most uplifting discoveries to emerge from this area of research is that you can develop into a more optimistic individual – in spite of the legacy of your genes, upbringing or experience of life. Things are more flexible than we might imagine. Fast forward two decades and now I'm a practising optimist and testimony to its many mood-enhancing benefits. I say 'practising' as it's something I still do consciously as a form of psychological self-defence. And that's why optimism is worth developing, because it acts as a shield that protects you from spiralling down into depression. I teach the techniques now to my clients and many times I've witnessed a palpable sense of relief when someone successfully defeats a monster of a pessimistic belief. Pessimism often grows to gruesome proportions, while optimism is more delicate and needs nurturing for it to develop.

How pessimism leads to depression

Pessimism puts you on a fast-track to depression, while optimism protects you from it – optimistic people are more resilient in dealing with life's stresses and able to bounce back easier than pessimists. If you are pessimistic about the chances of something working out, you're less likely to put in the effort to guarantee its success and more likely to give up when you hit an obstacle. This, of course, makes it even more probable that the bad thing you're dreading will go on to happen. It becomes a self-fulfilling prophecy. This is the essence of 'learned helplessness'.[2] You have a pessimistic belief that 'whatever I do doesn't matter' – there is nothing you can do to change or control a difficult situation and so you give up, lose hope and become helpless. Depression lurks in the shadows. Pessimists are also liable to ruminate as a way of responding to distress – to brood on the causes and consequences of the source of suffering, going over it endlessly again and again. People who have the habit of ruminating are more likely to become depressed.

Over 30 years of study has found that people with a pessimistic outlook are more vulnerable to depression and health problems. Pessimists are susceptible to learned helplessness, which is influenced by their 'explanatory style' – this is the manner in which you habitually explain to yourself why events happen. Having an optimistic explanatory style prevents depression, while a pessimistic explanatory style increases helplessness and this, in turn, can trigger depression. Martin Seligman found that by learning optimism you could improve an individual's mood and health.

Optimism – self-defence for the mind

Optimism is a way of thinking that relieves the negativity generated by pessimism. Optimists see the glass as half full. They expect good things to happen and have a sense of confidence about life working out well for them. In a nutshell the mechanism that makes optimism work for people is this. If you expect something to turn out well, you're more motivated to put in the effort to ensure that success happens. And because you put in the effort, it is *more* likely to happen. Optimists are more successful than pessimists in the workplace. When it comes to health, it is the optimists who enjoy greater psychological and physical well-being. They cope better when things go wrong and experience less distress, depression and anxiety. Optimists have better immune systems and recover faster from surgery – they also live longer. When bad news intrudes on an optimist's life, surprisingly they don't go into denial. They focus instead on finding a way of solving problems and that's why they adapt better to negative events. So, for example, they're more likely to go to the doctor to check out their symptoms and stick to health advice. The research confirms that the optimism about optimism is fully justified, as it's associated with many of the good things in life:

+ Happiness

+ Positive mood

+ Satisfaction with life

+ Good health

+ High performance

+ Success

Are there any disadvantages to optimism?

So far it sounds like optimists have all the advantages, but there are a few drawbacks:

+ Optimists sometimes lean toward an inaccurate perception of reality, which results in them becoming unrealistically confident.

+ They can see themselves as low-risk for certain diseases and may underestimate the health risks, for example, of smoking.

✦ They may be inclined to take part in high-risk activities such as speeding, drinking and driving, and casual sex.

Optimists can become vulnerable to stress when they deny their negative emotions or persist in striving in situations over which they have little control. One potential threat to an optimist's well-being is having their rosy view of life shattered by a serious trauma or loss. For a pessimist this would merely confirm their beliefs, but for an optimist it could lead to a breakdown in their worldview and a loss of confidence in their ability to influence events in their lives. However, the evidence suggests that optimists may be better equipped to rebuild their world. Pessimists are more likely to go into denial when there is a difficulty, whereas optimists are more likely to face up to it. Pessimists pay more attention to dealing with the difficult emotions generated by adversity, whereas optimists are more focused on dealing with the problem itself.[3]

What about pessimism?

I can hear some of you protesting that pessimism is more realistic: it's the safe option, you're less likely to be disappointed when things don't work out. If you're a pessimist, you probably know all too well how depressing it can be. Pessimism is a way of thinking that focuses on the negative, emphasizes problems and anticipates things going wrong. Pessimists expect the worst to happen and when it does, it confirms that they were right all along to think pessimistically. This then becomes a self-fulfilling prophecy, which reinforces a pattern of negative thinking. There is some evidence, however, to suggest that a mild dose of pessimism is not altogether a bad thing in old age. One study found that among the elderly, a realistically pessimistic perspective is associated with adapting better to negative life events.[4]

A positive in pessimism?

There is a form of pessimism that is more positive than most. If you are the type of person who is always prepared; who carries an umbrella in case it rains; who figures out all the alternative routes to get to your destination in case of transport strikes or who rehearses endlessly for a presentation you've delivered successfully many times before, then you are likely to be a 'defensive pessimist'.

Defensive pessimism is a coping strategy used to manage anxiety. What defensive pessimists do is to prepare for the worst. Think of it as being the embodiment of the scouts' motto 'Be prepared'. They set low expectations to help 'cushion' the potential blow of failure and play through various mental scenarios, paying special attention to all the possible things that might go wrong. They then work hard to prepare for the task ahead to avoid failure. And it generally pays off. If you recognize yourself in this, then take heart. Defensive pessimism seems to be a successful strategy for those inclined to worry. It helps you to gain a feeling of control and channel that anxiety into putting the effort in to perform well. Positives in this form of negative thinking if you are by nature a defensive pessimist is that it can lead to better performance, self-esteem, making progress toward goals and developing supportive friendships.[5]

Two different ways of thinking

The key difference between optimism and pessimism is in the way we explain things that happen to ourselves, our 'explanatory style'. These are the automatic thoughts that interpret the events that happen to us.

EXPLANATORY STYLES

We explain events in three ways:

| Me | Not me |

Always .... Not always

Everything .... Not everything

PERSONAL ... PERMANENT ... PERVASIVE ...

It's not so much what happens to you that counts, as the way you explain it to yourself. This is what marks the difference between optimistic and pessimistic thinking. So let's look at how a pessimist thinks when a bad event happens to them. This is their explanatory style:

✦ **It's me** (personal)

✦ **It's always** (permanent)

✦ **It's everywhere** (pervasive)

Here's an example of how a pessimist reacts in practice. Let's say they were unsuccessful at a job interview, they might think:

✦ It's all my fault. I was awful. They didn't like **me** (personal).

✦ It's **always** like this. I'll never get another job (permanent).

✦ This bad luck is **everywhere** in my life. It's all ruined (pervasive).

You can hear how painful it is when you're giving yourself such messages – that the misfortune is all your fault (personal), it's forever (permanent) and will blight everything in your life (pervasive). An optimist thinks in the opposite way to a pessimist. So when something bad happens to an optimist, they think:

✦ **It's not me** (not personal)

✦ **It's not always** (not permanent)

✦ **It's not everywhere** (not pervasive)

If we apply this explanatory style to the same scenario where you've been unsuccessful at a job interview, this is how it might sound:

✦ It's nothing to do with **me**, they must have found someone more experienced (not personal).

✦ It's not **always**, I've applied successfully for jobs in the past, I'll apply successfully for jobs in the future (not permanent).

✦ This bad news isn't **everywhere**. Other parts of my life are going well right now (not pervasive).

An optimist is thinking that it's just one bit of bad news that's not personal, only temporary and only in this particular slice of life. In this way an optimist is able to minimize the negative impact caused by a bad event.

Think like an optimist when things go wrong

If you're a pessimist, try experimenting next time something bad happens by thinking like an optimist – not me, not always, not everywhere – to minimize the pain and disappointment. There are three dimensions to this.

1. Think of the other possible causes for the bad thing happening. Rightly or wrongly optimists are more inclined to blame external causes (others, circumstances) for things going wrong rather than themselves (all my fault).* This helps to preserve their self-esteem.

2. Remind yourself that this is more likely to be temporary although it may feel permanent. Look to

*Although this is characteristic of how optimists think, you should still take resposibility for your life choices.

the past for evidence of things changing. We change, the seasons change, every cell in your body will change. This, too, will pass.

3. Look more broadly at other areas of your life. So you might have had a disappointment in this slice of life, but what are the other life areas that are currently working well? Think of home, work, relationships, health, finances, play, study, spiritual practice, etc.

Think like an optimist when good things happen

Optimists and pessimists also think in opposite explanatory styles when they're considering the positive events in their lives. When a good thing happens to an optimist, they think:

✦ **It's me** (personal)

✦ **It's always** (permanent)

✦ **It's everywhere** (pervasive)

So if something good happens such as having a successful job interview, an optimist would think that it was all down to them (personal) – their skills, their performance at the interview, their wow factor; that this good fortune is going to stay (permanent) and that it will have a beneficial effect on other areas of life (pervasive). For a pessimist it's the other way around when a good thing happens. They think:

✦ **It's not me** (not personal)

✦ **It's not always** (not permanent)

✦ **It's not everywhere** (not pervasive)

So, when the pessimists shock themselves by getting the job they went for, they believe that it was a fluke rather than anything to do with them (not personal), that the good fortune will run out (not permanent) and that it won't affect the rest of life, which is still bad (not pervasive).

	OPTIMIST SAYS	**PESSIMIST SAYS**
Positive Event	**Me:** The good thing is all down to me.	**Not me:** It's a fluke! Nothing to do with me.
	Always: This is here to stay!	**Not always:** It's just a one-off. It won't last.
	Everywhere: This good fortune is going to spread.	**Not everywhere:** But everything else is bad.
Negative Event	**Not me:** It's nothing to do with me.	**Me:** It's all my fault.
	Not always: This too will pass.	**Always:** It's for ever.
	Not everywhere: It's only this small area of life, other things are going well.	**Everywhere:** It's going to affect everything in my life.

Tune into your automatic negative thoughts

To change the way you think about things means con-sciously interrupting your automatic thinking. The first stage to becoming a learned optimist is to tune into this internal dialogue and the critical voice in your head, and to notice what automatic negative thoughts are playing on your internal radio station. You may begin to recog-nize the flavour of your pessimism. Are you someone who thinks that everything that goes wrong is your fault and ignores extraneous circumstances?

Or are you someone who thinks that when things take a turn for the worse that's the way it will stay. I worked alongside a self-confessed 'recovering pessimist', who flew in from the USA to facilitate a training programme and as a very tall American was unused to the fixtures and fittings of the standard British hotel room. The showerhead was set too low for him and he grouchily resigned himself to having to crouch down to use it. On day three he noticed a lever and lo and behold – the showerhead shot up! This is typical of the mundane way in which the permanence of pessimism shows up – you make an automatic assumption that something is fixed and can't change. Another manifestation of pessimism is when you over-react to something going wrong, imag-ining that it has ruined everything in your life rather than seeing it for what it is, that this particular part of life is under stress.

Learning optimism

The way we explain the things that have happened indicates the attitude we will take to events in the future and this affects our mood. People with a pessimistic explanatory style who suffer bad events are likely to become depressed, whereas people who have an optimistic explanatory style are much more resistant to depression. Martin Seligman describes ways of cultivating optimism in his classic book *Learned Optimism*.[6] Through the ABCDE model, he explains the process of how we think about the events in our lives and how to defeat pessimistic thinking using one of three Ds.

A = Adversity: 'A' stands for the adversity, the facts of what occurred.

B = Belief: 'B' is your belief about the adversity in the moment. This is your interpretation of what happened.

C = Consequences: 'C' stands for the consequences on your emotions and behaviour. These consequences are driven by your 'B', your belief about the adversity.

D = Disputation, Distraction, Distancing: 'D' represents the three methods positive psychology recommends to deal with the pessimistic belief.

E = Energize: 'E' stands for the renewed energy and relief when a pessimistic belief is successfully defeated.

Seligman recommends getting to know your ABCs so that you begin to recognize how it is your belief about what happens which drives the consequences for your emotions and behaviour. Carry a notebook in which you list the adversities that happen and later sit down and separate out the A from the B and the C. Use the example in the chart below.

A (Adversity) – A friend hasn't responded to the invitation to my birthday party

B (Belief) – She doesn't care about me

C (Consequences: how you felt and what you did) – I felt angry, upset and I deleted her from my address book

A (Adversity) – _____

_____

B (Belief) – _____

_____

C (Consequences: how you felt and what you did) –

_____

_____

The next bit involves tackling the pessimistic belief – the B – using one of the three **Ds – Disputation, Distraction or Distancing. Disputation** is the main tool here. Imagine you're a barrister in court, arguing with the pessimistic belief. Ask yourself these questions.

✦ What is the evidence for this belief? For and against?

✦ Is there an alternative explanation for what happened?

✦ What are the implications of holding this belief?

✦ How useful is this belief to me? Does it work for or against me?

The most powerful way of disputing a pessimistic belief is to show how it might be inaccurate and to do this requires evidence. Because the mind may be automatically seeking out evidence that confirms pessimistic beliefs, it is likely to miss out on the evidence that contradicts the belief. So, in the example above, while you're feeling low because of what you believe to be your friend's insensitivity in not responding to your invitation, maybe you're missing out on other evidence, for example that the friend is away on a trip and may not have received it.

By examining the evidence you may discover causes for the adversity that are neither personal, permanent nor pervasive. This can feel a little clunky in practice as you attempt to interrupt the automatic negative thoughts, but it is worth sticking with and persistence does make it easier. You may even become able to talk yourself down from the habit of defaulting to the worst possible outcome of what might happen, which is often the case with pessimistic thoughts as they spiral out of control. So in the example you might go from *'my friend's not answered my invitation and she doesn't care'* to *'none of my friends care'* to *'I don't have any real friends'* and then to *'no-one cares about me'*. All because one person has not responded to an invitation.

You can see how the pessimistic belief takes on a life of its own of monstrous proportions and how uncovering the evidence that your friend is away on a trip can short-circuit that catastrophizing. I do this frequently with coaching clients, looking at the evidence and helping them to interrupt their sprint to the worst possible outcome.

A variation on disputing the belief is to look for an *alternative* explanation for what happened, as there is often more than one cause for events. By generating alternative explanations, you may find a less personally destructive explanation – for example, that the friend hasn't seen the invitation rather than that no one loves me.

It's a similar story if you ask yourself what are the *implications* for holding that belief? So even if the pessimistic belief that you've been snubbed by this particular friend is true, what does that imply? You may have lost this particular relationship, but it doesn't mean that you've lost all of your friendships.

Finally, how *useful* is it to you to have this belief? Does it serve you? For instance, is it helpful to imagine that all your friends have abandoned you? Unlikely. All these techniques help you to interrupt the automatic flow of pessimistic thoughts and find a less damaging explanation for what's happened.

Alongside Disputation are two other **Ds** – **Distracting** and **Distancing**. Both of these are geared to manage the intensity of emotions such as fear, anxiety and anger that result from negative thoughts. When you regain your composure, you're more able to use disputation to tackle the pessimistic belief and find an explanation for the negative event that is less personal, permanent or pervasive. What do you use to distract yourself? It may be consciously putting your attention on something else. Or it could be removing yourself physically from the location you're in – maybe by going for a walk – or starting a conversation with someone. Distancing is similar to distracting, it's about putting some distance between yourself and the pessimistic thought so that it has less of an impact. What works well for you to distance yourself from negative beliefs?

A reframe – finding an alternative

Reframing is another technique that can be used to combat pessimism. It involves finding a positive in a negative situation. So, say you were planning a country walk one Sunday, but as the day dawned it was raining hard and the walk was cancelled. You ask yourself: how can I get something positive out of this? You could reframe it by seeing it as an opportunity to have a long lie-in or to head to a rural pub for Sunday lunch or to catch up with a DVD you've been wanting to watch. So, you find a positive in the negative, the disappointment of cancelling your walk. It takes some of the sting out of the negative situation. It may provide some consolation and, even if it doesn't, by learning to reframe you'll be acquiring the habit of challenging negative thinking and defending yourself against the bitter pill of pessimism. Here are some sample scenarios to reframe. See if you can find a positive for these negative situations:

+ You have a bad dose of flu and are stuck at home.

+ You fail your driving test and you can't retake it for another month.

+ You're the only one among your friends who is not in a relationship.

I've taught this technique to young people and found that it works particularly well as a first step in developing optimistic thinking. I remember one teenager I worked with who was living in a hostel but threatened with eviction, which would have made him homeless. He faced a very difficult situation but amazingly Sam* still managed to reframe it. He said that if he were evicted from the hostel, he'd be leaving a place he had little liking for and might be temporarily housed in a bed and breakfast where the breakfast would be free! Sam was evicted but ended up reunited and living with his mother, so his reframe may have helped him indirectly on the path toward a more positive outcome.

*Name changed

Is it possible?

I find a very useful question to develop optimism in the most entrenched of negative thinking is to ask: 'Is it possible?' So even if Sam had been deeply pessimistic about his situation, is it possible – literally – that he could end up in better accommodation? Yes, of course it is! Is it possible that someone can find new love after a loss? Yes, of course it is! Is it possible that someone can find employment after redundancy? Yes, of course it is! Is it possible that someone can be happy again? Yes, of course! You may struggle to believe it, but on paper all of these things are possible.

Women who worry – dames do depression

Depression is a feminine issue. Women tend to experience higher highs and lower lows than men and are twice as likely to experience depression, according to psychologist Susan Nolen-Hoeksema.[7] One of the reasons for this is rumination. Women are more likely to reflect on what's gone wrong, to chew over problems endlessly, analyzing obsessively, whereas men are more likely to distract themselves and take action. This rumination, paired with a pessimistic thinking style, leaves you vulnerable to depression. As well as over-thinking the past, women also tend to over-think the future, worrying about what might happen, imagining the worst. This can lead to distortions in thinking patterns, which can tip over into anxiety and depression and increase vulnerability to substance misuse.

The over-thinking trap

Here are some tips to manage worrying.

+ Distract yourself.

+ Write your fears down. Putting them on paper can take the heat out of them in your mind.

+ Avoid the triggers that set off over-thinking – specific places or situations.

+ Take one small step a day toward solving the problem. Before you know it, things will have moved forward.

TIME TO WORRY

This is an exercise for those who worry too much, are overemotional and prone to anxiety, depression and anger. The aim is to stop kill-joy interruptions to your day and save them instead for a specific time. This is useful when you find yourself 'sweating the small stuff' or struggling with things you have little control over.

→

- As soon as you notice yourself fretting over something, postpone the worrying by promising yourself that you'll think about the problem later in the day during a designated 'worry time'.

- Set aside 15–30 minutes for your 'worry time'. Choose a time when you know you'll be calm and collected, for example after some relaxing or physical activity.

- If you notice gremlins surfacing outside the 'worry time', try to distract yourself with a mindful practice (see Chapter 6), or some other activity such as physical exercise.

Based on Quality of Life Therapy[8]

We've looked at how optimism can be used to combat the negativity of pessimism, but you can also use optimism in its positive sense, to generate positive feelings about the future. Psychologist Laura King has found that writing about your 'best possible future self', creating a vision for your ideal life, has great benefits for psychological and physical health, including an immediate boost in positive emotions, an increase in happiness weeks afterwards and, over the longer-term, decreased rates of illness.[9] This is a grounded approach to creating an ideal vision of the future based on having goals rather than the stuff of sheer fantasy. People are instructed to consider their most cherished goals in each area of life and visualize what it will be like achieving those goals. Writing about your 'best possible future self' works well to promote optimism and generate an abundance of positive emotions, as well as the hope that fuels the drive to make these goals a reality.

If you're familiar with journaling, you may already have some idea as to why writing about your 'best possible self' works well. The act of writing down your vision helps you to gain insight about what's really important to you, your priorities in life and what motivates you. Plus, it can generate ideas of how to reach those goals and navigate around any obstacles in the way. In this version, from a study by psychologists Ken Sheldon and Sonja Lyubomirsky, people were invited to do the exercise as often as they felt like over the course of four weeks. So if you like journaling, writing or quiet contemplation, then this exercise could be a good one for you.

YOUR BEST POSSIBLE SELF

Find a peaceful, comfortable place to sit where you won't be disturbed.

Take 20–30 minutes to think about how you would like your life to work out for the best at a point in the future – 1, 5 or 10 years away. Think about your 'best possible self', imagine yourself in the future, after everything has gone as well as it possibly could. You have worked hard and succeeded at accomplishing all of your life goals. Think of this as the realization of your life dreams, and of your own best potentials.

Based on Sheldon & Lyubomirsky[10]

Sonja Lyubomirsky recommends this activity as a way of developing the 'optimism muscle'. Like any new habit optimism takes practice, so do persist with this and the other exercises and, as they become easier to do, you'll begin to see the brighter side of life and eventually this will be infused with a heart-felt positive emotion.

Hope for the best and prepare for the worst

As with everything in life, it is all about balance. Blind optimism can get you into as much trouble as total pessimism. Martin Seligman recommends a 'flexible optimism', which you choose to apply appropriately.

When to choose optimism

✦ When you're concerned about how you will feel – keeping your morale up or fighting off depression.

✦ When the situation will be protracted and your physical health is the issue.

✦ When it's about an achievement, such as gaining a promotion, selling a product or winning a game.

✦ When you want to lead, to inspire others, or to get people to vote for you.

When to choose pessimism

The guideline is to ask yourself what is the cost of failure in any particular situation. If the cost of failure is high – endangering life or important relationships, then choose the more cautious, pessimistic route. So, in the case of a drunken partygoer contemplating driving home, it is better to choose the pessimistic route and take a taxi. You'd prefer an airline pilot to apply pessimism and check out that funny sound in the engine before take-off.

Another psychologist, Sandra Schneider, suggests a hybrid combining optimism and realism, which she calls 'realistic optimism'.[11] This is about hoping and working toward the outcome you desire but tempered by a realistic outlook, so that you have an accurate view of the situation (rather than looking at it through rose-tinted spectacles) and you know how to proceed to achieve success. It is not about expecting that something will land in your lap without putting in the necessary effort.

A word to the wise on learning optimism

I don't want you to beat yourself up if you find it hard in your attempts to cultivate optimism. The thing about automatic negative thinking is that it is just that – automatic. The pessimism habit is a tough one to shift. Change certainly *is* possible, although questions remain over how large or permanent a change can be expected.[12] The advantages of optimism are such that every little bit counts. Be kind to yourself, keep going, don't judge your efforts and be grateful for every small step achieved. Even after 20 years I wouldn't claim to be a natural optimist, rather a learned optimist. Learning optimism is a life-long practice, but it is definitely worth it.

The one to read: *Learned Optimism: How to change your mind and your life* by Martin Seligman

CHAPTER 8

Resilience: The Road to Recovery

+ **What is it?** The ability to deal with tough times and bounce back from them

+ **Try this for:** Coping positively with adversity, moving forward after a setback

+ **If you like this, try also:** Positive Emotions (Chapter 3), Optimism (Chapter 7) and Vitality (Chapter 10)

Breakdown, loss, conflict, bereavement and ill health are a few of the adversities that we may endure in a lifetime. Life is full of challenges, stress and suffering – it's an inevitable part of the human condition. But whereas some people go under when faced with a crisis, others are able to sail through life's tough times and bounce back from them. This is because they are resilient and like happiness, resilience can be developed.

So far in this book we've looked at positive psychology techniques that are geared toward promoting your well-being. This chapter focuses on ways of recovering your well-being after a setback, a trauma or a loss. Resilience is about being able to deal with life's adversities and overcome them. A colleague of mine describes resilience as like the water level in a reservoir. Imagine you're in a boat and there are rocks ahead representing rocky times – a difficulty or a crisis. If your resilience (or water level) is high, then you're more likely to sail over those rocks unscathed. But if your resilience (or water level) is low, then you're more likely to hit the rocks.[1]

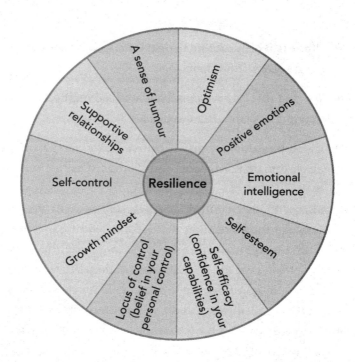

The question is how to fill your reservoir with well-being so that you build resilience. There are plenty of ingredients that contribute. Developing any of these will raise your level of resilience and help you to avoid being tossed about by the stormy waters of life.

Resilience is one of the major areas of positive psychology, equipping people to reach for a positive outcome in difficult circumstances. This focus on resilience shows how positive psychology tackles the negative by asking questions, such as what are the positive ways of coping with difficulty? What works to support your ability to bounce back? And is there anything positive to be gained from your negative experiences? We'll look at what helps in this chapter.

Ordinary magic

The good news about resilience is that it doesn't require extraordinary capabilities. Instead, it relies on ordinary skills such as being able to come up with a realistic plan. Ann Masten, one of the experts in the field, calls it 'ordinary magic'.[2] As well as enabling us to bounce back from life's harshness, resilience also operates as a form of protection against the ill-effects of stress. Some resilience skills develop in childhood, but you can also pick them up as an adult. Karen Reivich and Andrew Shatté from the University of Pennsylvania have identified seven core ingredients in psychological resilience, all of which can be developed.[3]

1. Emotional awareness and regulation

This is the ability to identify which emotions you're experiencing and have some control over how you feel.

2. Impulse control

Resilient people don't rush into things, they can control their impulses and put up with uncertainty.

3. Optimism

Optimism (*see* Chapter 7) is possibly the most important resilience skill you can develop. Pessimism undermines resilience.

4. Causal analysis

Being able to think through why things happen and consider problems from different perspectives.

5. Empathy

Being able to understand the emotions of others. This helps you to build relationships and gain two-way support.

6. Self-efficacy

This is about having confidence in your ability to solve problems and using your strengths.

7. Reaching out

This is the ability to reach out to others, but it's also having the will to take calculated risks and accepting when things don't work out.

Positive Coping

When a crisis hits, your first line of defence is your habitual coping style. People generally use one of three forms of coping – emotion-focused coping, problem-focused coping or avoidant coping.[4] It's worth getting to know which style of coping you favour because there are advantages and disadvantages to each, as you can see in the chart overleaf.[5]

Emotion-focused coping is when your attention is on dealing with the emotional distress caused by the crisis, rather than on resolving it. Not every crisis has a solution to it, of course, nor is it within our control – such as in the case of a bereavement – so finding a way to deal with the pain might be the sensible option. Emotion-focused coping includes talking things through with a confidante or counsellor, the emotional release of crying and drawing on support from friends and family.

What often works well is to attend to overwhelming emotions first and then when you feel calmer and have a clearer head, you'll be in a better position to make plans and move forward. This is the essence of **problem-focused coping**, where your attention is on what steps you can take to resolve the issue. It's a more active form of coping, appropriate for calamities in which you can exercise some control, such as in the case of a business failure. By taking on the responsibility and coming up with a plan of action, you have a map to help you move forward. While it's important to manage the emotions involved, eventually it will pay off to develop more of

Emotion-focused coping	Problem-focused coping
POSITIVE	**POSITIVE**
Processing emotions	Accepting responsibility
Talking things through	Developing a realistic action plan
Leaning on friends for support	Seeking accurate information
Crying – emotional discharge	Using optimism
Exercise and relaxation	
NEGATIVE	**NEGATIVE**
Seeking meaningless support	Procrastination
Taking the stress too seriously	Developing unrealistic plans
Alcohol and drug abuse	Not following through on strategies
Embarking on destructive relationships	Pessimism
Aggression	
Unproductive wishful thinking	

a problem-focused strategy, so that you can pick up the pieces and begin the journey forward.

The third style of coping, **avoidance-coping**, is as the name suggests – about blocking the crisis out and engaging in distractions. Denying the existence of a problem sounds like an all-around negative, but in the short-term it can serve a positive purpose as a distraction that can help you rally yourself before tackling the issue. This depends on choosing a healthy distraction, such as seeking out social activities rather than something unhealthy, such as drowning your sorrows in drink. Over the long term, though, you are better off facing up to the issue and finding a way of managing it rather than turning a blind eye and risking things getting worse.

Take a moment now to identify your usual style of coping. Think back over the last crisis you had to cope with. What did you do? Was your focus on dealing with the emotions, solving the problem or on distracting yourself from the pain?

✦ If your style is emotion-focused, try coming up with an action plan to take you forward.

✦ If your style is problem-focused, consider whether you might need some emotional support to address how you feel about the crisis and help your recovery.

✦ And if your behaviour is avoidant, then take a deep breath and turn your attention to what's going on. What actions could you take to improve your situation?

The ABC of resilience

I advise coaching clients to focus on building resilience on three levels – targeting their thinking, emotions and physical selves. You've already had a preview of the main thinking technique used in resilience – the ABCDE that features in the previous chapter on optimism. The key component here is to understand how your thinking operates when something difficult happens. Here's a reminder:

✦ When an *Adversity* happens …

✦ You have a *Belief* or thought associated with it, which is your interpretation of what happened. This *Belief* leads to …

✦ *Consequences* for your emotions and behaviour – how you felt in that moment and what you did, even if you did nothing.

The important thing to note is that it is the beliefs rather than the adversity that drive the consequences. The adversity is simply the facts of what's happened. One person's minor irritation is another person's calamity, because they have different beliefs in play about the adversity. Resilience is about taking control of the parts that you can change. You may not have much control over the adversity, but you can influence your beliefs about it and that is the bit we target. It's not so much what happens to us that counts but more the way we think about it, because it's our interpretation of what happens that drives the emotions and behaviour that follow on from it. So, to give you a simple example:

You're stuck in traffic (the *adversity*) and your *belief* might be that you're going to be late and lose your job (notice how these thoughts default to the worst possible outcome) and the *consequence* might be that you feel anxious (emotion) and take a risk attempting an illegal shortcut (behaviour).[6]

The first stage in resilient thinking is to become familiar with your own ABCs. After an adversity occurs (especially the small ones that can be easier to make sense of), note the thoughts and beliefs that you had in the moment and the consequences for your emotions and behaviour. You will probably begin to notice that some emotions crop up more frequently than others. This is your feedback mechanism that gives you a clue as to what types of beliefs are in play.

Some people find it easier with strong emotions to work backward – to identify the consequences first and then work out what was the belief or thought driving those emotions. An example of that might be arriving home one evening to a note from the postman saying that he was unable to deliver a parcel and experiencing a fit of anger (the consequent emotion). Working backward you might discover that the anger (the C) was generated by a belief (the B) that your Saturday would be ruined by having to go and collect the parcel.

Fill in your own ABCs in the chart overleaf. (I have put in an example to show you what to do.)

Adversity	Belief	Consequences
(What happened – the facts)	*(Your interpretation)*	*(Emotions and behaviour)*
Bumped into neighbour's car	He's going to hate me!	I felt nervous (emotion) and avoided him (behaviour)

Once you get into the habit of breaking down your ABCs, you may begin to notice how the patterns in your thinking lead to anxious, sad or angry feelings. This is valuable information in itself because it can reveal your dominant tendencies, whether it is to anxiety, depression, anger, etc. It is these repetitive negative thoughts and emotions that undermine resilience and can trigger the downward spirals into depression.

Tackling these negative beliefs involves challenging how we think about adversity and adopting more healthful ways of thinking. The good news is that you've already seen most of these techniques in the chapter on optimism (pages 111–136) with the D of disputation. *The Resilience Factor*,[7] the positive psychology guide to resilience, describes this as encouraging *accurate* and *flexible* thinking. Accurate thinking is about weighing up the evidence that supports or challenges the beliefs that we hold. Flexible thinking is about being more malleable in the way we think, coming up with alternative and more optimistic ways of looking at the situation. You may wonder why we don't just do this as a matter of course. What gets in the way is the perilous pair of the **confirmation bias** and the **negativity bias**.

The **confirmation bias** is the habit we have of seeing the evidence that supports our beliefs and ignoring evidence that doesn't. So, we notice everything that fits with our view of the world and miss all the clues that contradict it. If the negative belief is that you'll never get another job following redundancy, you'll notice all the evidence that seems to support that, such as the economy being in recession. And you'll ignore the evidence that contradicts that belief, such as more people being in work than are out of work even when the economy is depressed.

This is where the negativity bias teams up with the confirmation bias. The brain leads you to focus on what's wrong, such as sad stories of being out of work, and so you ignore the tales of success of those for whom redundancy marks the start of an exciting, expansive chapter of life.

If you are depressed, your mind will be supplying you with all the evidence that confirms your depressing view of the world, which can plunge you deeper into the downward spiral. Knowing that these biases exist is helpful, but that's only part of the story because there are all kinds of tricks the mind plays on us – mistaken assumptions and thinking errors that we are likely to fall into when we're stressed or depressed. These all hamper our ability to think flexibly. Taking a step back to observe your thoughts (mindfulness is great for this) will reveal how the brain operates, taking the negative on trust and mistrusting the positive.

Aaron Beck, one of the pioneers behind CBT, realized that this 'distorted thinking' is linked to depression. Feeling low is driven largely by how we think about the world. By interrupting these automatic thoughts we can stop ourselves being sucked into the downward spiral. Opposite is a list of some of the most common thinking errors. See if you recognize the ones you generally fall prey to.

All these thinking errors are common, especially in

depression, and give you a blinkered view. As this distorted thinking is automatic, this is another reason to work through the ABC of events so that you can begin to see which of these thinking errors might be in play, affecting your thoughts.

THINKING ERRORS[8]

- **All-or-nothing thinking** This involves thinking in absolute terms. 'Things are *always* going to be like this'. 'It *never* changes'. All-or-nothing thinking is a key player in depression. Challenge it directly: 'Always? Never? Is that really the case?'

- **Mental filter** These are the grey-tinted glasses on life. Focusing almost exclusively on one small element of an event, usually the most upsetting or negative part.

- **Magnifying and minimizing** Distorting reality by magnifying the negative in a situation (making a mountain out of a molehill) or minimizing the good.

- **Dismissing the positive** This consists of continually running down or diminishing the positive aspects of a situation.

- **Jumping to conclusions** Leaping to conclusions (usually negative). This can take the form of 'mind reading', where you make assumptions about what someone is thinking or 'fortune telling' where you anticipate how things will turn out.

→

- **All about me** Thinking that you are the cause of all the misfortune that happens around you.

- **All about you** Blaming others and circumstances for adverse events and being blind to your own role.

- **Overgeneralization** Taking isolated examples and turning them into rules of how the world operates.

- **Emotional Reasoning** Making decisions based on feelings rather than objective evidence.

- **Should statements** Inflexible patterns of thinking about how the world 'should' be, how others 'should' behave.

- **Labelling** Putting a negative label on people and events, for example labelling someone as a loser.

Externalizing the negative belief by writing it down or talking it through with someone can help to distance you from the brain's mental trickery. You may not even realize that your beliefs are so negative, believing instead that they are simply factual – for example. 'I've lost my job, I'll never get another job'. By writing it down, you can spot more easily that this is a piece of all-or-nothing thinking, and challenge it. By examining the evidence you can separate the facts from the beliefs and begin to recognize your negative thinking patterns. Below is an example of someone cross-examining a negative belief. Have a go with some of your own beliefs. This is a way of testing the accuracy of your beliefs and challenging the negativity.

Adversity: My relationship broke up.
Belief: I'll never be in a relationship again.
What's the Evidence?

- I've been in relationships for more years of adult life than I've been out of one.

- People form new relationships after divorce. I know X and Y (specific evidence) have gone on to have new relationships.

- You can form relationships at any age; for example, there are stories of senior citizens falling in love and long-lost loves finding each other.

Adversity:
Belief:
What's the Evidence?

....

....

....

....

....

....

....

→

Adversity:
Belief:
What's the Evidence?

....

....

....

....

Adversity:
Belief:
What's the Evidence?

....

....

....

....

Adversity:
Belief:
What's the Evidence?

....

....

....

....

I find the question, 'Is it possible?' (that we met in the last chapter, *see* page 130) really useful here. So, is it possible that you could form a new relationship? Unless you live in a highly repressive regime that bans relationships, the answer is most definitely yes!

The deep well of resilience – your positive emotions

Positive emotions also have a role to play in our deeper resilience. They undo the effects of negativity and stress, and act as protection against depression, helping you to bounce back from negative experiences. Studies examining the aftermath of 9/11, a time of great stress in the USA, showed that the presence of positive emotions amid the negativity accelerated the physical recovery from the trauma and helped people to find meaning in negative situations.[9]

Think of how laughing can lift the mood in the darkest of times. Humour is an example of something that generates positive emotions and helps people to deal with adversity. By seeking out joyful experiences that put sunshine in the soul, you'll feel better and build resilience. Positive emotions loosen the grip of negativity on your mental outlook. Barbara Fredrickson, the expert on positive emotions, suggests that positivity lies at the heart of resilience, putting the brakes on the slide into depression. Moments of gratitude and other positive emotions enable you to regain your perspective, reverse the downward spiral and bounce back.[10]

Being able to tap into positive emotions marks the difference between people who experience stress reactions that dissipate fast and those for whom stress escalates and lasts for days. And this happens on a physiological level too. Positive emotions act as a 'reset button' helping the body back into the parasympathetic nervous system, returning the heart rate and blood pressure to normal. It's not that resilient people don't experience negative emotions, it's just that they're better able to accommodate positive emotions alongside them. All the preceding chapters contain activities that will help you to fill that reservoir of positive emotions to raise your level of resilience.

For first-aid resilience, think physical

Resilience-thinking techniques require a calm mind, something that can be elusive in the middle of adversity. Physically, our bodies may be on full alert, experiencing the 'fight or flight' physiological reaction with the release of stress hormones such as cortisol and adrenaline. The amygdala (the part of the brain associated with stress, anxiety, fear and anger) is aroused. This is all counter-productive to the calm, rational thinking needed to manage the adversity, which is why in the heat of the moment it often pays off to look at what you can do physically to calm your body down. By doing this your body switches from the red alert of the sympathetic nervous system (which prepares us for fight or flight) into the calm of the parasympathetic nervous system (the rest-and-digest response), which helps us to calm down and to access a quieter place to think straight.

Resilience first-aid kit

✦ Deep breathing

✦ Any physical activity, for example – walking, jogging, dancing, swimming

✦ Meditation

✦ Yoga

✦ Martial arts, such as tai chi

As well as serving as a first-aid kit, the body also plays an important role in your underlying level of resilience. Think of how your ability to cope is compromised when you're tired, run-down, ill or not sleeping well. And how good sleep, decent nutrition, physical activity and abundant energy can help you to see things in a more positive light. Your physical well-being influences your resilience, so respect the mind–body connection and remember how tending to your physical body will support your mental ability to deal with the adversity.

Reaching out

Sometimes it's only when we hit rock bottom that we finally find a way out of depression. A positive in hitting rock bottom is that this is often the moment when we begin to reach out to others. So often we try to soldier on alone until we reach a point where nothing seems to be working. On a personal note it was only when I hit rock bottom and ground to a halt that I noticed so much kindness and compassion in others, even strangers.

One of the ingredients of resilience is to reach out. There will be people who want to help you out of the dark tunnel into the light , so pluck up the courage and reach out to them. You may be pleasantly surprised by who turns out to be your angel of resilience. There is a community in depression, of other people who've been through the bleakness and understand what it's like. Support is not only to be found in people you know, there are also self-help support groups that can help, such as the Depression Alliance[11] in the UK. Sharing your experience with others who have faced similar challenges can help you on the road to recovery.

Heroes of resilience

Other people can also be a source of inspiration. Do you have a resilience hero? Do you know someone who has overcome adversity and gone on to thrive? It could be stories of people who've come through crises, such as the

Chilean miners trapped deep underground; or political leaders who survived periods of imprisonment, such as Nelson Mandela in South Africa and Aung San Suu Kyi in Burma; or sporting heroes, such as the cyclist Lance Armstrong, who triumphed over cancer to win the Tour de France a record seven times; or even historical figures who displayed great resilience, such as Anne Frank. Then again, it could be someone closer to you.

Another way of developing resilience is by learning from the successful strategies of resilient people. Who can you take inspiration from? What did they do to survive and thrive? I have a friend who reads books about great feats of endurance when she's down, such as on people who've sailed the world single-handedly or survived kidnap. This is comforting as well as inspiring, as the misfortune she endures rarely matches what she reads about in the books.

WHO IS YOUR RESILIENCE HERO?

1. What challenge did they face?

2. What strengths did they show to get through?

3. What strategies did they use to get through?

4. What can you learn from their experience?

Remember, too, that you might be your own resilience hero. Think back over your hard times. How did you deal with them? What were the lessons you learned then that might help you with the difficulty you may be facing now?

Finding a positive in the negative

People experiencing challenging times sometimes speak of finding unexpected benefits in their negative experiences.[12] These benefits include discovering a greater meaning in life, having better relationships, finding a capacity for empathy and forgiveness and a sense of wisdom and are related to better physical and psychological health. To give you some examples, in one study people whose homes were destroyed in a fire experienced positives, such as the helpfulness of others and learning important life lessons. People who lose a loved one to a long-term illness can sometimes experience stronger family bonds and a new perspective on life. It would be insensitive of me to encourage you to ignore the negative consequences of the adversity in favour of searching for benefits. However, knowing that there are potential gains for your mental health further down the line, do try to appreciate any positives that emerge amid the sea of negativity.

Beyond resilience: post-traumatic growth

It may surprise you to learn that even in life-shattering events where things are never the same again – the death of a loved one, a natural disaster, acts of terror or war, a terminal diagnosis or a life-changing injury or illness – there can still be positives. Not only do we have the capacity to bounce back from adversity, we can also develop positively as a result of it. This is a phenomenon called **post-traumatic growth** – positive changes that occur as a result of attempts to cope in the aftermath of traumatic life events.[13] This is not about denying the suffering or offering some kind of token consolation. Even in the worst of life events a hint of something positive can emerge. Enlightenment and growth can co-exist with trauma and despair. The positive can exist alongside the negative. Here are some of the benefits reported by people who've experienced post-traumatic growth.[14]

✦ A 'better self'; feeling stronger – 'if I can get through this, I can get through anything'; feeling more alive, more authentic and more open to what life has to offer; increased confidence, competence and independence; greater maturity and humanitarian instincts.

✦ Stronger and closer relationships with people; a greater appreciation for others and realizing who your true friends are; increased love, empathy and compassion for others; more of a sense of community and a greater ability to relate to others, particularly fellow trauma survivors.

✦ A greater sense of meaning in life; a fresh appreciation for the preciousness of life itself; a new and wiser philosophy on life; enhanced spiritual awareness; a shift in priorities to what's really important to you; a fresh sense of appreciation for all the good in one's life.

Post-traumatic growth is something that occurs organically rather than being something we can induce. It tends to happen in traumatic, life-changing events that shatter our view of the world. There are two ways in which we can react to such events – **assimilation** and **accommodation**. Think of a beautiful vase that breaks into pieces. You can glue it back together again. It will look more or less the same, but have more cracks and be more fragile than it was before. This is what happens in assimilation. You try and integrate the trauma into your current worldview.

The other thing that you can do with a broken vase is to take the pieces and create something new out of it, maybe a piece of art such as a mosaic. So the vase is turned into something new and potentially more solid than the glued-together vase. This is accommodation, where you modify your worldview to accommodate the reality of what's happened – and this is what can give rise to post-traumatic growth. Rather than focusing on rebuilding life exactly how it was before (assimilation), the aim is to build a life that will work within the new situation (accommodation). So, someone who is widowed is more likely to experience post-traumatic growth if they can find a way to adjust to being single. Positive accommodation in the case of trauma involves accepting that random negative events can happen and there is nothing you can do but to try and live with the here and now as successfully as possible.[15]

Writing about adversity

One thing that can help to reveal the hidden benefits within adversity is to write about it. Putting distressing experiences into words is a form of catharsis, helping to get them off your chest, make sense of your experiences and find some kind of meaning in them.[16] It also helps to organize your thoughts so that you're more likely to come up with ideas about what to do. James Pennebaker is the psychologist who has studied the therapeutic properties of writing about adversity. Although it can be upsetting in the moment as you relive what's happened, over the longer-term even a short spell of writing about adversity for 15 minutes a day over four days has advantages for health, such as better immune-system functioning and improved performance. One study carried out with a group of engineers who'd gone through the trauma of redundancy showed that the act of 'expressive writing' led to positives that included increased offers of new employment. So in this particular case, writing about adversity helped with resuming employment after unemployment.

ADVERSITY JOURNALING

Want to give it a go? You may already be familiar with journaling, used as a personal development tool to process thoughts, gain insights and tap into creativity, such as in Julia Cameron's *The Artists' Way*. The idea here is to write in free-form, without stopping and without regard for the niceties of spelling, grammar, etc. Aim to keep going for 15 minutes at a time.

Over the next few days, I'd like you to write your very deepest thoughts and feelings about one of the most traumatic experiences of your life. In your writing, I'd like you to really let go and explore your emotions in depth. You may link your experience to your relationships with others. You may also want to link it to your past, your present or your future, or to who you have been, who you would like to be, or who you are now. You can write about the same general issues or experiences on all the days of writing or about different traumas each day.

Based on James Pennebaker[17]

The ones to read: *The Resilience Factor* by Karen Reivich and Andrew Shatté

Resilience: How to Navigate Life's Curves by Positive Psychology News

CHAPTER 9

Positive Connections: Other People Matter

✦ **What is it?** Relationships are the leading source of happiness

✦ **Try this for:** Happiness, positive emotions and life satisfaction

✦ **If you like this, try also:** Savouring (Chapter 4) and Gratitude (Chapter 5)

When it comes to our happiness it is beyond all doubt that 'other people matter'.[1] We are social creatures with a deep need to connect and that includes relationships with friends, family, colleagues, even pets. We become happier when we think in terms of 'us' rather than 'me'. A defining characteristic of the top 10 percent of happy people is that they have good close relationships and lead active social lives.[2] Many of the activities that build happiness and well-being involve other people. One of the most effective ways of deepening the joy of a positive experience is to share it. This chapter explores some of the many ways in which you can nurture the relationships in your life and spread a little joy by taking happiness from the personal into the inter-personal.

As human beings we have a fundamental need to belong. A sense of belonging generates positive emotions and the reverse is true, too – losing that sense of community leads to negative emotions. One of the ways in which depression takes us into a downward spiral is by isolating us. We don't feel much like being around others and yet having social contact provides a source of support, as well as a distraction from negative thoughts. People who are alone or feel alone suffer more mental illness than those with more social connections.

Many a song has been written about it and the science of well-being agrees that love, in all its forms, really does make the world go around. People who prioritize love over money are happier than those who put a premium on wealth. I remember one workshop in particular with a group of young people. During a discussion over what does and doesn't make us happy, I told them that wealth plays only a limited role in happiness and once your basic needs are covered, money ceases to have much of an effect on well-being. This was such a head-on clash with their beliefs that there was nearly a riot! For them money *was* the route to happiness. I then got them to do an exercise which involved savouring their happiest memories. Out came all these wonderful stories about falling in love, the births of babies and special times spent with loved ones. And that's when they got it – they realized that none of their cherished memories came with a price tag attached. The best things in life really are free. Having the knowledge that happiness is more likely to be found in relationships than in bank accounts, gives you a strong clue as to where to invest your efforts to increase your well-being. Prioritize the people in your life. Spend time with them. Cherish them.

Nurturing relationships

Relationships are coming under increasing strain in the 21st century with the focus on the individual rather than the collective. We tend to favour the 'me' over the 'we', whereas earlier generations put a greater emphasis on the needs of family and society. Martin Seligman links the epidemic in depression partly to this trend toward individual satisfaction.[3] One of the symptoms of depression is self-absorption. Focusing exclusively on the self in an attempt to 'find happiness' can backfire and be a route to disappointment. We know that happy people tend to experience a greater sense of the 'we'. Given that relationships are so key to our well-being, it is certainly worth finding ways to nurture your personal connections. You'll realize why relationships require so much care when you read this next bit!

The positivity ratio in relationships

Just as we have a positivity ratio for us to flourish as individuals, there is also a positivity ratio for relationships and it stands at 5:1, higher than that for individual well-being. That means it takes five positive experiences (such as being affectionate, kind or interested in what's going on in each other's life) to make up for every negative event (such as being hostile, critical, ignoring your partner or hurting their feelings). Negativity is highly destructive in relationships, with more potential to inflict damage on a relationship than the positive has the capacity to heal and unite a pair. This positivity ratio comes from the research of John Gottman, who has studied relationships for many years in his 'love lab'[4] and has been able to predict with great accuracy which couples will stay together and which will break up, based on the way they interact with each other. Incidentally the positivity ratio in couples that divorce is typically under 1 : 1, so they rate marginally higher on negativity than positivity.[5]

Of course, you could end up taking this in literal fashion and the next time you fall out with your partner, make it up to them not only with an apology (1), but also with wine (2), meals (3), treats (4) and ... I'll leave the rest to your imagination! But joking aside you can see how corrosive negativity is for a relationship if it requires so many positive things to compensate for its ill effects. Gottman rates the top four most destructive emotional reactions within a relationship as defensiveness, stonewalling, criticism and contempt. Be warned!

Five good things

The negativity bias that makes us notice what is wrong before we see what is right also influences relationships. So you are more likely to pay attention to your loved ones' vices than you are their virtues. One way to counteract this negativity and to nurture your relationships at the same time is to actively remind yourself of someone's positive points, whether it's their kindness, loyalty, energy, sense of humour, work ethic, etc. This can also mean the good things that they've done – times when they might have helped or supported you. Gratitude helps relationships to run smoothly, to become aware of the give and take and to appreciate what you receive. Aim to record five positives about your loved one to nudge you in the direction of the positivity ratio.

WHAT I LOVE ABOUT ....

1. ....

2. ....

3. ....

4. ....

5. ....

Let's talk actively and constructively

Psychologists agree that the way you communicate is critical for the success of any relationship. There are four main styles of communication in a relationship according to Shelly Gable, only one of which is beneficial for the relationship.[6] This is revealed by the way we respond to positive news. See if you can identify your own style in the examples below of responses to good news. Then, check out the style used by others you know and notice any patterns in your way of responding.

The good news	Typical response	Way of responding
I've got a new job!	'OK, that's nice' (low-key)	PASSIVE and CONSTRUCTIVE Quiet, low energy support
I've got a new job!	'You know, my back's really playing me up today.'	PASSIVE and DESTRUCTIVE Ignoring the good news; changing the focus to yourself
I've got a new job!	'What about that extra stress you'll be taking on?'	ACTIVE and DESTRUCTIVE Quashing the good news

→

The good news	Typical response	Way of responding
I've got a new job!	'That's really great! Is it the one you wanted? When do you start?'	ACTIVE and CONSTRUCTIVE Enthusiastic support, asking for details; leads to capitalizing

Based on Gable *et al*[7]

Active Constructive Responding is a way of reacting to someone's good news with enthusiasm and energy rather than in a passive or destructive manner. By giving someone your full attention and asking questions, you prompt the holder of the good news to think of even more positives and this enables them to truly savour the good that's happened, to capitalize on their positive event. It's the only style that builds the connection and turns a good relationship into a better one. There are gains on both sides – increased positive emotions, happiness, self-esteem and decreased loneliness. The relationship itself benefits with increased satisfaction, liking, intimacy, trust, commitment, closeness and stability.

All the other forms of responding have a negative impact on relationships. This includes Passive Constructive, which seems positive but because it is such a limp, low-key response, it leads to an energy mismatch where the high energy of the good news is dampened by the low energy of the response. The next time you are on the receiving end of someone's news, notice how you react.

✦ Do you help them to savour their good news?

✦ Does their high energy find a match in yours?

✦ Do you build the positivity between you or break it?

Social emotions

Emotions are contagious. They spread rapidly through groups, workplaces and organizations. This holds true for both positive and negative emotions. A joyful mood can be infectious, passing from one person to another, but equally so can a mood of gloom or anxiety, bringing everyone down. So, not only can your personal mood spiral up or down, so can the mood of the group around you. This is something to be aware of, especially if you are easily affected by other people's moods, as many sensitive people are. If you work or associate with people who are constantly moaning, the negative mood will catch hold and spread. The brain has 'mirror neurons', which fire off in response to observing emotions in others.[8] What this means is that we pick up emotions from others not only because we observe them, but also because we experience them directly as these mirror neurons fire. This is the reason why I choose to watch comedies on TV to catch the infectious humour and avoid the diet of depressing news.

Use this knowledge to spread delight rather than despair. Instead of perpetuating pessimism, point out the positives in any situation and try to overcome the collective negativity within groups. Although they are fleeting experiences, the effects of positive emotions accumulate, so you have the potential to make a beneficial impact on the mood of your groups. Here are some thoughts to help you to manage the contagious nature of emotions.[9]

+ Smiling is infectious. Smile and pass your good mood on.

+ Other people matter, but avoid being drawn into other people's misery. You can be compassionate without joining in.

+ Identify who are the 'radiators' and the 'drains' in your life. 'Drains' are the people who suck the energy out of you, whereas 'radiators' are people who give out warmth and whose company is energizing.

+ Create 'high-quality connections' in your workplace.[10] These are based on a mutual positive regard, trust and active engagement on both sides. Any point of contact with another person is an opportunity for a high-quality connection, where people feel engaged and open, which in turn increases energy and the likelihood that people will help each other.

+ Protect yourself from 'corrosive connections' – poor-quality connections that sap the energy in an organization. These are based on distrust and a lack of regard. It can be hard to avoid corrosive connections if they come in the form of a boss. Try not to take it too personally – it might simply reflect a lack of social skill in the other person.

The how-not-to of social comparisons

One of the barriers to well-being is that we humans have a toxic tendency of comparing ourselves to others. Am I as successful? As happy? As attractive? As rich? As slim? This sense of competition runs deep as we tend to judge our own opinions and aspirations by comparing ourselves to others and this has a profound effect on how we rate ourselves.[11] Social comparisons affect us in all kinds of ways and can lead to us making irrational choices. For instance, studies have found that people would rather take a lower salary and earn more than their colleagues than have more money in real terms but less than their teammates. The perception of whether we're earning more or less than our colleagues has a bigger effect on our well-being than the amount we're actually earning.

If you're depressed then social comparisons are the ultimate feel-bad experience. You're more likely to feel wounded if you judge yourself to be lacking in some respect compared to someone else. This then generates a noxious brew of negative emotions, such as envy, resentment, anxiety, sadness, anger or disgust, combined with low self-esteem and insecurity. Happy people are more likely to rise above self-punishing comparisons. They still make comparisons, but other people's triumphs have less of an effect on their well-being.

Compare down not up

Upward comparisons are to people we perceive to be better off than we are. This can be a source of inspiration in some circumstances – when the other person's success is within your grasp. Then, it can fuel your motivation and drive to achieve something similar. However, upward comparisons are frequently made to people who are not within reach, such as celebrities with their perfect-looking lifestyles. Such upward comparisons can leave you feeling inadequate and down.

It's best to distract yourself from making unfavourable comparisons, but if you can't there is an alternative, which *does* help your well-being. That is to compare yourself downward to people who are less fortunate than you. It sounds like a rather dubious thing to do, but it does work. Comparing downward can help you appreciate what you've got. It's a great antidote for the poisonous stew of negative emotions generated by unfavourable upward comparisons. So, for example, I compare myself to people living in politically unsettled, poor nations and this also has the added benefit of making me grateful that I live in a stable democracy.

Cherish the love

The old adage that 'love is the best medicine' holds a lot of truth. If relationships are the primary source of happiness, then to love is the ultimate strategy that builds well-being. Love is a multi-faceted feature of positive psychology – both a strength and a positive emotion. Moments of love are made up of a whole host of other positive emotions, from joy and gratitude to serenity, hope, pride, amusement, inspiration and awe.[12] And the more of these you experience, the more likely you are to experience a sense of 'oneness' with other people, so that your sense of self expands to be more inclusive of others, changing from 'I' to a greater sense of 'we'.

If social comparisons are toxic for your well-being, then love is most certainly the tonic. Love comes in many forms from romantic love, which matures into a more companionable love, to love for children, parents, family and friends and a wider love, such as for humankind and the planet. Cultivating love in your life and recognizing it when it appears is a powerful way to build your well-being. Cherishing love is a form of savouring (see Chapter 4). By savouring the love in a relationship you can deepen the benefits of love. One way of doing that is by voicing your appreciation of the love you share. One long-term study of marriages shows that communicating the savouring of love to a spouse has a beneficial effect on the quality and resilience of the relationship. Bryant and Veroff offer tips on savouring a romantic partnership, which could equally be applied to developing the bonds in other types of relationships.[13]

✦ Share interests and activities

✦ Pay close attention to the details of their life so that you appreciate their likes and dislikes

✦ Collaborate on a shared task

✦ Disclose things about yourself to promote intimacy

Sharing is not only good for relationships, it also strengthens the benefits of savouring. In fact sharing the savouring is one of the most reliable ways of raising the level of enjoyment on offer. Think of how you might share some of the activities in the book. For example, you could make the 'three good things' exercise (*see* page 82) something you do with a friend or partner and experience happiness bouncing back and forth between you.

Acts of kindness

The more you give the more you receive. Acts of kindness are total win:win actions because not only do they help others to feel good but they help you to feel good, too. Altruism is just as beneficial for your psychological health as it is for your relationships. Acts of kindness are about performing good deeds for others, whether it's offering support to someone in need or contributing your time to a worthy cause. Volunteering is often put forward as a remedy for the blues. It is a way of distracting yourself from your own problems and from rumination, one of the risk factors for depression. Kindness is also a positive emotion, so practising it will help you to move toward the positivity ratio of 3:1 positive to negative emotions and into an upward spiral to greater emotional well-being. Being kind to others increases your own happiness and lowers levels of stress and negative emotions.

Acts of kindness can be spontaneous or pre-planned. What works well, according to experiments conducted by Sonja Lyubomirsky, is to inject variety into what you do to keep the kindnesses fresh and meaningful and to concentrate the acts into a short period of time. This intensifies the power of kindness to boost your mood.[14] But a word of warning – your good deed needs to originate in a genuine desire to help. If you feel coerced or obligated for whatever reason, then the benefits of kindness are limited both for yourself and for the person on the receiving end.[15] Your motivation needs to be intrinsic (kindness for its own sake) rather than extrinsic (kindness for an external reward).

Performing random acts of kindness for complete strangers has evolved into a social movement in recent years, spreading joy and promoting global well-being. A similar idea is to 'pay it forward', to do good deeds for others in recognition of having yourself been the lucky recipient of some unconnected kindness. If you're looking for inspiration for your own acts of kindness, there are plenty of ideas on websites associated with this worldwide phenomenon.[16]

Forgiveness

If you're wondering what forgiveness is doing here, it's because forgiving others for the harm they have done you is good for *your* personal well-being. Letting go is healing. The benefits of forgiveness are that it reduces depression, anger, anxiety and feelings of hostility, as well as helping your physical health by reducing stress and blood pressure.[17] I know it is easier said than done but if you can view it as something you're doing for yourself rather than for the other person, you'll no longer be drinking from the toxic cup of negative emotions that a lack of forgiveness produces. Forgiveness is an antidote to resentment, anger and dark thoughts of vengeance. Even though the wish to retaliate is strong, by giving into the desire for revenge, you risk setting up a vicious cycle of escalating acts of harm. Forgiveness is not the same as condoning, excusing, forgetting or denying the harm that has been done. Neither is it about being a doormat to someone's abusive behaviour or restoring the relationship with the other person. It's about responding to transgressions with mercy instead of vengeance. You don't have to have contact with the transgressor in order to forgive. You could write a letter of forgiveness without sending it. Forgiveness is evolving into a social movement with groups that bring together victims with the perpetrators of harm to help the victims to heal, freeing themselves of the hurt caused and moving forward with their lives.[18] In positive psychology forgiveness is recognized as a strength of character. By developing this strength, you can gain the virtue of temperance.

Virtual friends

Recently I was home alone suffering with flu. I felt miserable and lonely. I posted a status update on a social media website and within hours a stream of messages of support had been posted on my 'wall'. It was like the sun coming out after a grey day. My mood lifted. I was alone but no longer lonely.

It's very easy to question whether these 'virtual friends' count as real friends. I prefer to think of it as a way of opening yourself up to a new horizon of social interaction and to view it as an addition to, rather than as a substitute for, face-to-face socializing. Social media can give you a great sense of connectedness as long as it's not at the expense of real-life connections. Through social media I am able to stay connected to friends in different parts of the world, to keep up with events in the lives of friends both near and far, to make connections with people who have the same special interests and to be part of a global community in my field. And some of these 'friends' are people I've never met but have been able to connect with online.[19] However, you won't be surprised to hear that there is a limit to the number of people in your life with whom you can maintain a meaningful relationship. What you may not know is that the number stands at around 150, according to evolutionary anthropologist Robin Dunbar.[20] This is the maximum number of social contacts that you can sustain in your personal community and still have some kind of quality within the relationship.

Appreciate your weak ties

Although it is the small number of our close relationships – the supportive strong ties – that hold the most value for our well-being, there is also something to appreciate in the quantity of our wider acquaintances. Weak ties are those people we don't know so well, acquaintances who exist more on the periphery of our lives. You might think that many of your social media connections are weak ties, of little meaningful value compared to the strong ties in your life. However, in certain circumstances weak ties can be more beneficial than strong ones.[21] The theory goes something like this. Whereas our strong ties tend to move in the same circles as we do, weak ties move in different social circles, so they provide a bridge into new circles of people, resources, even jobs. So a network of social media friends, for example, can open up all kinds of new possibilities. This is the strength of weak ties and a reason to value those connections.

Married, single, other …

I'm aware that a lot of this chapter reads as if couples win hands down in the happiness stakes and that single people fare badly. While it is true that getting married is one of the few things that can increase your set point for happiness, the picture is not as straightforward as it appears. For starters the initial boost in well-being does tend to wear off eventually, although overall happiness levels are higher for the wed than the unwed. It is, however, the quality of the relationship that counts; being in a bad marriage is worse for your well-being than being single or divorced. Co-habiting couples also do well in terms of their happiness, although not quite matching the advantages of being in a good marriage. So, a secure, stable, successful marriage tops the league in terms of the benefits for well-being.

Single and divorced people are, according to studies, lower on happiness than their married or co-habiting counterparts. One of the reasons for this is because of the lack of readily available psychological support. After a rotten day at work, sharing your woes over a glass of wine helps to alleviate the stress and this is more difficult if you're living on your own. The answer if you are not in a close, personal relationship is to build those supportive networks around you. I've lived both the life of a singleton and the attached. The support I give and receive from my female friends is just as valuable as that gained from a partner. The difference is that you have to work that bit harder to develop those support networks rather than relying on having support on tap from a partner.

Our faithful friends

When it comes to getting over the black dog of depression, your pet may also have a role to play. There are many health benefits from interacting with pets. I have friends who attribute their recovery from depression to getting a dog. Here's a flavour of what they say.

'Having a dog made me feel better because I had a dependent, the dog needs you to take it out and feed it. The dog gives you love and you have something to love in return. Dogs are upbeat, enthusiastic and when your dog is wagging its tail looking forward to the next thing, you can't help but be taken somewhere else in your mood.'

'I can honestly say that getting my dog was a significant part of healing for me, after my father died. I had lost interest in the world, gained lots of weight, lost confidence and stopped socializing. Getting Sabbi ensured I had to walk her outside each day, which had a twofold benefit: it connected me to nature which was very nourishing and it got me exercising again, so I gradually started to lose the weight and gain a desire to interact with the world around me again.'

'What I realized was that getting a dog helped me not to fall back into depression. I had to look after something. It's the responsibility that made the difference. I've got to look after somebody else and so I have to look after myself.'

'It was kindly pointed out to me that my lurcher, Bob, is in fact my longest male relationship, currently running at 10 years! Not only is he loyal, dependable and trustworthy, he is kind and loves me 100 percent unconditionally. Of course he helps with my well-being!'

~

With social isolation on the rise, dogs seem to have a particular role to play in forging connections that enhance your well-being – my friends can barely get around the park without half a dozen conversations with fellow dog-walkers. Having a dog is social, it distracts you from ruminating over what's wrong and develops fitness through all those walks. It can even lead to a relationship – I know a couple who met through their pets and are still together 20 years later!

+ Dogs help safeguard against depression

+ Owning a dog can reduce stress and anxiety

+ Owners who walk their dogs are healthier than non-dog owners

+ Owning a dog reduces blood pressure

+ Dog owners make fewer visits to their doctors

+ Owning a dog boosts your immune system

+ Dog owners are likely to recover faster from heart attacks

The research confirms that owning a dog has benefits for both physical and psychological health.[22] Scientists in Japan report that dog owners get a surge of the 'love drug', the bonding hormone oxytocin, when playing with their pets, which dampens stress and combats depression.[23]

One to read: *Social Intelligence: The New Science of Human Relationships* by Daniel Goleman

CHAPTER 10

Vitality: Mind, Body and Spirit

+ **What is it?** The holistic nature of well-being

+ **Try this for:** Energy, positive emotions

+ **If you like this, try also:** Meditation (Chapter 6) and Positive Directions (Chapter 12)

Human wellness is holistic. It's about the interconnections between mind, body and spirit (meaning in life). This chapter is about the other elements that influence your happiness. Psychology can sometimes give the impression of being a science that ignores what's going on beneath the neck, such as the impact that the body has on the mind and how the physical affects the psychological. Good mental health is built on the foundations of physical well-being. Sleep, diet, exercise, relaxation – all of these things have a knock-on effect on whether you feel up or down. When you lack meaning in life, you are more likely to feel down. When your energy is low, you're more likely to feel low. Physical illness depresses the mood and chronic or serious health problems leave you more vulnerable to depression. The good news is that the body can also work as a positive to support your psychological well-being.

The first-aid kit

When you're down it can seem like it might take a super-human effort to summon up a glimmer of an optimistic thought or connect with the slightest of positive emotions. This is where physical activity comes in handy. By moving physically your body produces endorphins, feel-good hormones, which lift your mood naturally. And as your mood lightens, you're more able to think in positive ways. That's why I regard physical activity as the first-aid kit, a way of kick-starting your upward spiral toward greater well-being on the back of a release of endorphins. This helps you into a better mental space, which then supports putting into action the strategies described in this book.

The challenge is to find a form of physical activity that you can persuade yourself to engage in. Depression drains energy, which makes it hard to be motivated to move physically. So set your sights on something small and manageable. That might mean something as simple as a short walk down the road, dancing around your home to music (even three minutes can have a positive effect) or five minutes outdoors working in the garden. Notice how your mood begins to shift as you do something physical. Movement works on other levels, too. It's a distraction from brooding and also a source of creativity. Moving physically can result in shifting mentally. If I'm stuck trying to figure something out, I find that I am able to solve it as I walk.

The key is to find an activity that you enjoy, that feels like a pleasure rather than a punishment. What works best for you? Here are some ideas:

+ Walking

+ Swimming

+ Cycling

+ Jogging

+ Yoga

+ Martial arts

+ Gardening

+ Dancing

I would choose the last item on the list – dancing is the fastest route I know to a mood boost. For one of the first happiness researchers, Professor Michael Argyle, it was Scottish country dancing, which he additionally rated for its benefits of being social and to music – two factors that also lift the mood. A clue as to which physical activity to choose is to think of what puts you into 'flow', that pleasant state of immersion, where you lose track of time. In sports it's often referred to as 'being in the zone', but you can also find it in activities such as gardening or tai chi.

Physical activity has a positive effect on brain chemistry. It's a natural anti-depressant with many benefits for your emotional health.

Physical activity ...

✦ Boosts mood through the release of endorphins

✦ Alleviates stress and anxiety

✦ Increases self-confidence and a sense of control

✦ Distracts from negative thoughts and emotions

✦ Encourages social interaction

The health guidelines for treating mild-to-moderate depression in the UK include the recommendation to take exercise. Physical activity can also stop you from relapsing into depression. One American study compared the effects of exercise, anti-depressants and a combination of both on people with major depression. All the groups showed significant improvements, but six months after the experiment ended, the people who had recovered in the exercise group had significantly lower relapse rates than those in the medication group. Continuing to exercise reduced the likelihood of a further diagnosis of depression. Exercise is one of the best forms of depression treatment.[1] It also has one advantage over psychological approaches because it requires little thinking beyond that required to get you engaged with doing it.

Green exercise – physical activity outdoors in nature – is particularly good for mental health. Even just five minutes of exercise in a green space boosts well-being.[2] I found that walking daily in my local park was tremendously helpful in beginning the journey out of depression and is something I've continued doing to this day. Here are some hints to make physical activity a part of your recovery:

✦ Make it **easy**. Go for small steps, rather than attempting something too ambitious, which might be too big and stop you doing it again.

✦ Make it **every day**. Incorporate physical activity into your daily life; walk instead of drive; take the stairs; turn the housework into a workout.

✦ Make it **sociable**. Find an exercise buddy – by having someone alongside you, you have twice the motivation to draw upon. It's also an opportunity to socialize, which is another powerful way of shifting your mood.

✦ Make it a **habit**. Exercise for someone who is prone to depression is rather like a daily shot of insulin for a diabetic – something you need to do every day but which is, ultimately, a lifesaver.

Rest and renewal

Do you remember when people had 'spare time'? When Sundays were a day of rest rather than a day to catch up? We live now in a 24/7 society where the boundaries between work and play have become blurred. You're never really off duty. Even the holidays are no longer sacred. Smartphones and laptops mean that you're always accessible, even when you're sitting on a beach. The 21st century barely acknowledges the need for rest and renewal. It's a way of life that is out of kilter and risks disturbing the balance of the mind.

I remember that my first experience of depression came after a long period where I was regularly working 60-hour weeks as a radio producer. On the outside I was successful, but on the inside I was severely stressed, on the go all the time and surviving on a diet of caffeine and sugary snacks. If I wasn't at work, I was thinking about work. I never switched off and eventually the inevitable happened – I burned out and succumbed to depression. When you ignore the body's need for renewal, you risk becoming depleted. Life becomes empty and flat. Classic signs of burnout are low mood, feeling disillusioned and a lack of energy. Unhappiness grows. The door opens to depression.

Pause for renewal

Rest may be an unfashionable word in our fast-paced modern society, but without it there is no renewal and you risk your mental health. Maintaining a balance between activity and renewal is important as too much of either leads to sub-optimal living. One thing that helps is to tune into the body's messages, which let us know when things are getting out of balance. If you have too much of one thing and not enough of something else, you'll hear a voice of complaint inside. Listening is about paying attention to your needs, whether it's for rest, renewal or more variety in life. It's easy to disregard these messages – this came home to me even in the process of writing this chapter alongside the day job. I was ignoring signs that life was getting out of balance until I was stopped in my tracks by an injury, which triggered an illness. That's when I finally got the message, except by then, of course, it was too late – my physical downturn in health was followed by a psychological one. I wish now that I'd paid attention to those messages telling me to rest and renew.

It helps to think of the body as having two main divisions to the nervous system and to consider how much time you spend in each. The sympathetic nervous system controls the stress response, which primes us for action and for 'fight or flight' when we face a threat. This is the adrenaline mode that pumps you up so that you can perform in the moment. The trouble is that many of us live our lives stuck in the sympathetic nervous system. The modern workplace depends on it. The parasympathetic nervous system, on the other hand, operates the 'rest-and-digest' response and other processes that happen when the body is in a state of relaxation. This is the route to renewal. What proportion of your time do you spend in the parasympathetic nervous system? Is there a balance?

If you've crashed and burned out, then your body is probably shouting at you to take it easy for a change. Renewal involves attending to your needs, restocking your reserves whether by resting, sleeping, good nutrition, physical exercise, getting out into nature, taking a break, doing something different or having a change of scene. All these things will also help to build your energy.

Energy: the fuel of happiness

Energy is a precious resource in the 21st century, not only in terms of the fuel that powers our world, but also the personal energy that enables us to engage with life. And engagement is, according to Martin Seligman, one of three routes to happiness alongside pleasure and meaning. Energy and emotions tread a similar path. High energy is often matched by a high emotion, such as joy. Conversely, when your energy is low, your mood tends to follow suit. Feeling depressed, hopeless or defeated are all states that are low in both emotion and energy. One of the characteristics of depression is the way in which it strips away every ounce of energy, leaving in its place a state of lethargy, from which it is hard to muster any kind of motivation to do anything.

Energy is in many ways the opposite of depression. Whereas depression depletes us of positive emotions, energy provides the fuel for happiness. It is useful, therefore, to understand more about the nature of energy. One principle of energy is that it diminishes both with overuse and underuse. You need a balance between expending energy and renewing it. Unfortunately, the need for recovery is often viewed as a sign of weakness rather than as a way to sustain performance. Loehr and Schwartz, authors of *The Power of Full Engagement*,[3] suggest that we think of energy as a series of sprints rather than as a marathon. A sprinter will engage powerfully for a short period, have their eye on the finishing line and then they'll rest before their next exertion. But a marathon runner keeps going until they drop. Loehr and Schwartz's recommendation is to live your life as a series of sprints – fully engaging for a period of time and then disengaging for renewal before jumping back into the arena. Another principle of energy is that you need to stretch it beyond your normal limits to build it up. This is how you develop the 'muscle' for energy, developing strength and flexibility as you go.

I noticed this happening when I turned to swimming to help my recovery from depression. The first steps were simply to get myself to the pool with the greatest of ease. That meant taking the easy route of driving myself there and committing to no more than getting into the pool. It is important to aim to do something small rather than setting the bar so high that it puts you off trying again. Having discovered that it was actually quite enjoyable to go for a swim, each time I pushed myself to do an extra lap. Very soon I was able to increase the distance I could swim and my vitality grew. The key is to make it really easy so that you actually do it, take the time to recover and then stretch yourself a bit further. You can develop 'muscle' in other areas, too, such as optimism. For example, the more you practise exercises such as the 'best possible self' (*see* page 133), the stronger and more authentic you will eventually become in your capacity for optimism.

As well as physical energy, there is also emotional, mental and spiritual energy. These can be built up in the same way that you build physical energy. So, stretch each type of energy beyond its usual limits – by then its functional capacity will be reduced, but after a period of recovery, it will be stronger than before and more capable of handling the next challenge. All these forms of energy share the same characteristics when they're functioning well: they have strength, endurance, flexibility and resilience. They are all connected, too, and take us into downward or upward spirals. So an energy-draining scenario might be one where you feel pessimistic about the future of the job you're in (emotional energy-drainer), and you waste a lot of time worrying about it (mental energy-drainer), so you comfort-eat mindlessly (physical energy-drainer), and so on downward.

An example of an upward spiral could be when you start walking to work and feel better for it (physical energy-booster) and your increased physical well-being then leads to you feeling more optimistic about life (emotional energy-booster). With this increased energy you begin to think more creatively about ways in which you can improve your work situation (mental energy-booster) and as you put them into action, you discover a new direction, which gives you greater meaning in life (spiritual energy-booster). You're into a virtuous cycle where one form of energy stimulates another.

Food for mood

It's a simple equation: what you eat has an effect on how you feel. Just as good nutrition improves your physical health, it also supports your emotional well-being. Your diet can have a positive influence on brain chemistry. It is neurotransmitters such as serotonin, the feel-good chemical, that tend to be out of balance in a diagnosis of depression. Serotonin affects the mood, and low levels of it are thought to be implicated in many cases of depression. A healthy diet will help you to feel better and build your vitality. The message is a familiar one – a nutritious, balanced diet contains lots of fresh fruit and vegetables (at least five a day), as well as lean proteins and complex carbohydrates. Consider including vitamins and other supplements in your diet, as the soil that produces our food is increasingly depleted of essential nutrients. Consult a dietician or nutritionist for advice tailored to your individual needs. Here are some insights on how you can munch your way to greater mental well-being.

Eating for happiness: feed the brain

✦ **Vitamin B** The B-complex vitamins are essential
for mental and emotional well-being. These are the
vitamins to counter depression, but the bad news
is that they can't be stored in the body so you need
to make sure they're in your daily diet or take a
B-complex supplement. **Folic acid** (aka **Vitamin
B$_9$**) is found in leafy vegetables such as spinach and
broccoli and is used to fortify cereals and bread.
Good sources of **Vitamin B$_6$** include meat, fish,
wholegrain produce, vegetables, nuts and bananas.
Vitamin B$_{12}$ is found in eggs, dairy produce, meat,
poultry and fish.

✦ **Vitamin C** Keep up your intake of Vitamin C, which
is known to be a mood elevator.

✦ **Serotonin** This is a feel-good chemical in the brain,
a neurotransmitter that regulates moods. To make
serotonin, the body needs **tryptophan**, an amino
acid. Tryptophan is present in most protein-based
food. You find it in poultry, red meat, fish, eggs,
beans, peanuts, seeds, oats, yogurt, cottage cheese,
chickpeas, bananas and chocolate (don't get too
excited – chocolate's benefits lie in a *moderate*
consumption of the 70 percent dark chocolate
variety). **5-HTP** (5-hydroxytryptophan) is another
amino acid involved in the production of serotonin,
which is available as a dietary supplement.

✦ **Complex carbohydrates** These have a calming effect. Carbohydrates provide the energy that fuel the body and they also help to produce serotonin. Your brain experiences a mild tranquilizing effect when you eat carbs – think of how comforting a plate of pasta or potatoes is when stress levels are high. Carbs calm the nerves, which is why many people turn to them when depressed or anxious. They are nature's chill pill. Choose **complex carbs** such as wholegrain pasta, bread, brown rice, legumes and beans that release their energy slowly for a longer-lasting effect.

✦ **Simple sugars** These stress the body. Refined carbohydrates are those found in many processed products, in sweet foods and those made of white flour, such as bread, cakes, pastries and biscuits. What happens is that you get a spike in blood sugar levels; eating **refined carbs** produces a sugar high, but then this is followed by crashing into a low, as insulin rushes to deal with the excess of sugar. This can leave you feeling even worse than before, with a drop in mood and energy. Fast-releasing sugars also stimulate the release of cortisol, a stress hormone, into the bloodstream.

✦ **Caffeinated drinks** Caffeine works by stimulating the central nervous system – often too much, especially if you are sensitive to it – which aggravates anxiety disorders, interferes with sleep, increases levels of the stress hormone cortisol and causes rapid fluctuations in blood-sugar levels. These are all factors that can worsen the symptoms of depression. Many people regard caffeine as a pick-me-up, but for people who are prone to depression, it can make the symptoms worse so it is advisable to cut back on it.

✦ **Water** The brain is about 85 percent water. Optimal brain functioning depends on having enough hydration to keep the brain signals moving. Water supplies energy to the brain; its cells require more energy than most other cells in the body. Water also facilitates the movement of the feel-good neurotransmitters serotonin and dopamine and removes feel-bad toxins from the body. The brain has no way of storing water, which means there's a risk of dehydration if you don't drink water regularly, so drink, drink, drink! Dehydration is associated with fatigue and negative moods – some experts believe there to be a link between dehydration and depression.

Laughter therapy

Something happens to people as they grow up. They become more serious as they take on adult responsibilities and the lightness and joy of childhood is lost. The laughs become few and far between. Laughter is a powerful way to bring that lightness back. As well as its ability to change your mood in an instant, laughter has benefits for physical health, too – lowering blood pressure, increasing tolerance of pain and boosting the immune system. Laughter is also a good stressbuster – simply anticipating having a laugh can stimulate the production of mood-boosting endorphins. You can enjoy the therapeutic benefits of laughter through watching comedies, seeking out social opportunities with friends who make you laugh or engaging in 'laughter yoga', a practice originating in India where people come together to participate in laughter exercises.

Spiritual well-being

Whatever your religious persuasion, if any, there is evidence to suggest that those who have a spiritual practice of some kind enjoy greater levels of hope, optimism and general well-being. They cope better in hard times and benefit from higher levels of emotional support when the chips are down. Having a spiritual practice can provide you with meaning in life and a sense of connection or oneness with something bigger than the self. A moment of contemplation brings peace and tranquillity into a busy world.

Meditation, the Eastern spiritual practice, has many benefits for well-being (*see* Chapter 6). Research shows that people regularly attending a religious service of some kind have greater well-being than those who don't, although this may be to do with the social support available through the faith community.

Spirituality can become more important in life as we grow older and wiser about what brings meaning to our lives. Spirituality also develops after experiences of trauma and depression. I use the word 'spirituality' as a non-denominational term, because this is not about any particular branch of religion. Some people find solace in the faith they grew up with, others gravitate to a spiritual practice that fits their personal values, some shop around in the spiritual supermarket adopting the parts that most appeal to them. For some a sense of spirituality is found in being close to nature, for others it is in a like-minded community. There is no doubt, though, that the spiritual – just like the physical – contributes to your psychological well-being, and both are elements to consider in your journey out of depression.

The ones to read: *The Power of Full Engagement* by Jim Loehr and Tony Schwartz

The Chemistry of Joy by Henry Emmons with Rachel Kranz

CHAPTER 11

From Strength to Strength: You at Your Best

✦ **What is it?** Your natural talents and positive character traits

✦ **Try this for:** Energy, positive emotions, well-being and success

✦ **If you like this, try also:** Positive Directions (Chapter 12)

Depression is an enfeebling experience – it leaves you feeling weary, with an overweening sense of your weaknesses. It's no surprise then that it is very easy to forget you also have strengths, and that these strengths can support you on the journey out of depression. Your strengths are your greatest assets, they are the clue to the real you. They point you toward a direction in life that is right for you (more on which in the next chapter). Your strengths strengthen you. They provide you with the fuel to power your life. People who actively use their strengths are more confident, happy, energetic, productive, resilient and satisfied with life. They enjoy greater well-being and success. Your strengths are the key to realizing your potential in life – they relate to the side of well-being that is about functioning well. The cherry on the cake is that when you use your strengths, you're on your way to excelling with ease because it's something that comes naturally to you!

Positive psychology is often referred to as the science of strengths, because they relate to the positive side of our characters – the things we're good at, our talents rather than our shortcomings. This is in contrast to mainstream psychology, which had become largely a science of human deficits prior to the arrival of positive psychology. Psychologist Alex Linley describes strengths as enabling optimal performance that is authentic and energizing.[1] You know you're drawing on a strength when you perform well in a task and the experience energizes you. Energy marks the difference between a strength and learned behaviour, which are things that you're good at but don't energize you. So you might be good at project management, but unless it's energizing for you then it isn't a strength. Another clue that you might be using a strength is when you find yourself going into flow ('in the zone') or thinking that 'this is the real me'. Your strengths hold a treasure trove of benefits for your well-being[2] because they:

✦ Generate optimism

✦ Develop confidence

✦ Encourage insight

✦ Produce positive emotions

✦ Provide a sense of direction

✦ Build resilience

✦ Protect against mental illness

✦ Help to achieve goals

An early experiment in positive psychology highlighted two techniques that work well to increase happiness and reduce symptoms of depression over the long-term.[3] One was finding new ways of using your strengths and the other was the gratitude technique, 'three good things' (*see* page 82). Using your strengths sets up a virtuous cycle – you perform well, which in turn generates positive emotions, overcomes the negativity bias and puts you on track for success. The benefits of using your strengths accumulate and can help you to move from a state of languishing into flourishing. One of the core principles of positive psychology is that your greatest potential for growth lies in developing your strengths rather than in fixing your weaknesses. So this is where to focus your efforts to get the maximum return.

People are often reluctant to talk about their strengths, preferring to focus on their shortcomings instead. Many of us find it hard to even recognize our personal strengths. If there's something we're naturally good at, we tend to assume that everyone else must find it easy, too. Not true! We tend to downgrade our strengths rather than take a pride in them. Your self-esteem will develop as a result of investing in developing your strengths – it helps to build confidence and overcomes a negative self-image.

The virtuous cycle of strengths

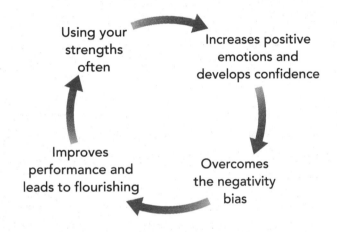

Using your strengths often

Increases positive emotions and develops confidence

Overcomes the negativity bias

Improves performance and leads to flourishing

Activating your strengths

✦ Begin a list of your strengths. Include positive character traits such as kindness, compassion, fairness, a caring nature, common sense, responsibility, leadership skills, etc.

✦ Add the things you're naturally good at and that energize you or put you into flow, such as writing, music, cooking, nurturing people or plants, etc.

✦ Ask friends and relatives what they think your strengths are.

✦ Return to the list whenever you think of something to add.

✦ You might want to keep the list in your journal or some other place where you can savour your strengths.

✦ When you have your list aim to use your strengths more. Choose a particular strength each day or week, and put it into action.

✦ Once you've made a habit of using your strengths, look for new opportunities in which you can apply them. This is the route to a sustainable increase in well-being.

How to identify your strengths

Now that you are aware of the merits of getting to know your strengths, it's good to get into a mindset of spotting strengths in yourself and others as you go about life. Here are some further clues to help you to identify when your strengths might be in play.

STRENGTHS-SPOTTING CHECKLIST[4]

Your Best: What are you doing when you are at your best?

Ease: What do you find easy and what are you naturally good at?

Energy: When do you feel at your most alive? What energizes you?

Authenticity: What makes you say 'this is the real me'?

Fast Learner: What sort of skill do you pick up rapidly and effortlessly?

Motivation: What do you do just for the love of it?

Focus: What are you naturally drawn to? What attracts your attention?

Flow: What puts you 'in the zone' where you're completely absorbed and lose track of time?

Passion: What are you passionate about? What are you animated talking about?

Childhood: What were you good at as a child? How does it show up in your life now?

A guide to human strengths

> Bravery, integrity, compassion, persistence, humility, forgiveness, fairness, gratitude, open-mindedness ...

Wouldn't it be great if there were a guide to all of humanity's positive characteristics? A guide that focused on what is right with people rather than what is wrong? One of the major achievements in positive psychology has been to create such a book, categorizing all the strengths that are valued across the planet. The *Character, Strengths and Virtues*[5] handbook and classification is the result of an ambitious collaboration between two of positive psychology's leading figures: Chris Peterson and Martin Seligman. They embarked on the mammoth task of surveying positive character traits across research, history and in different fields and cultures and then distilled them into 24 distinct character strengths, all of which are universally valued. It's like a manual of mental wellness. In effect it is the opposite of the *DSM* (the *Diagnostic and Statistical Manual of Mental Disorders*), the handbook that psychiatrists refer to in diagnosing mental illness. Each strength belongs to one of six groups or 'virtues' – wisdom, courage, humanity, justice, temperance and transcendence. By developing a strength, you can acquire whichever virtue that strength is linked to. So, for example, if you have character strengths of creativity, curiosity, love of learning, open-mindedness or perspective and you invest in developing them, you will gain the virtue of wisdom. If you have a strength in kindness or love, then you can develop the virtue of humanity. The chart below (pages 207–211) lists the 24 universal character strengths. As you read through them, notice when you recognize one of your own strengths.

THE VALUES IN ACTION (VIA) CLASSIFICATION OF CHARACTER STRENGTHS

WISDOM and **KNOWLEDGE** – cognitive strengths that entail the acquisition and use of knowledge

- **Creativity** (originality, ingenuity): Thinking of novel and productive ways to conceptualize and do things; includes artistic achievement but is not limited to it

- **Curiosity** (interest, novelty-seeking, openness to experience): Taking an interest in ongoing experience for its own sake; finding subjects and topics fascinating; exploring and discovering

- **Judgment and Open-mindedness** (critical thinking): Thinking things through and examining them from all sides; not jumping to conclusions; being able to change one's mind in light of evidence; weighing all evidence fairly

- **Love of Learning**: Mastering new skills, topics and bodies of knowledge, whether on one's own

→

or formally; obviously related to the strength of curiosity, but goes beyond it to describe the tendency to add systematically to what one knows

- **Perspective** (wisdom): Being able to provide wise counsel to others; having ways of looking at the world that make sense to oneself/others

COURAGE – emotional strengths that involve the exercise of will to accomplish goals in the face of opposition, external or internal

- **Bravery** (valour): Not shrinking from threat, challenge, difficulty or pain; speaking up for what's right even if there's opposition; acting on convictions even if unpopular; includes physical bravery, but is not limited to it

- **Perseverance** (persistence, industriousness): Finishing what one starts; persevering in a course of action in spite of obstacles; 'getting it out the door'; taking pleasure in completing tasks

- **Honesty** (authenticity, integrity): Speaking the truth but more broadly presenting oneself in a genuine way and acting sincerely; taking responsibility for one's feelings and actions

- **Zest** (vitality, enthusiasm, vigour, energy): Approaching life with excitement and energy; not doing things half-heartedly; living life as an adventure; feeling alive and activated

→

HUMANITY – interpersonal strengths that involve tending and befriending others

- **Love** (capacity to love and be loved): Valuing close relations with others, in particular those in which sharing and caring are reciprocated; being close to people

- **Kindness** (generosity, nurturance, care, compassion, altruistic love, 'niceness'): Doing favours and good deeds for others; helping them; taking care of them

- **Social Intelligence** (emotional intelligence, personal intelligence): Being aware of the motives/feelings of others and oneself; knowing what to do to fit into different social situations; knowing what makes other people tick

JUSTICE – civic strengths that underlie healthy community life

- **Teamwork** (citizenship, social responsibility, loyalty): Working well as a member of a group or team; being loyal to the group; doing one's share

- **Fairness**: Treating all people the same according to notions of fairness and justice; not letting feelings bias decisions about others; giving everyone a fair chance

- **Leadership**: Encouraging a group of which one is a member to get things done and at the same time maintaining good relations within the group;

→

organizing group activities and seeing that they happen

TEMPERANCE – strengths that protect against excess

- **Forgiveness and Mercy**: Forgiving those who have done wrong; accepting others' shortcomings; giving people a second chance; not being vengeful

- **Modesty and Humility**: Letting one's accomplishments speak for themselves; not regarding oneself as more special than one is

- **Prudence**: Being careful about one's choices; not taking undue risks; not saying or doing things that might later be regretted

- **Self-Regulation** (self-control): Regulating what one feels and does; being disciplined; controlling one's appetites and emotions

TRANSCENDENCE – strengths that forge connections to the universe and provide meaning

- **Appreciation of Beauty and Excellence** (awe, wonder, elevation): Noticing and appreciating beauty, excellence and/or skilled performance in various domains of life, from nature to art to mathematics to science to everyday experience

- **Gratitude**: Being aware of and thankful for the good things that happen; taking time to express thanks

→

- **Hope** (optimism, future-mindedness, future orientation): Expecting the best in the future and working to achieve it; believing that a good future is something that can be brought about

- **Humour** (playfulness): Liking to laugh and tease; bringing smiles to other people; seeing the light side; making (not necessarily telling) jokes

- **Religiousness and Spirituality** (faith, purpose): Having coherent beliefs about the higher purpose and meaning of the universe; knowing where one fits within the larger scheme; having beliefs about the meaning of life that shape conduct and provide comfort

Used with permission of the VIA Institute on Character © 2011

You may be interested to know that people who've recovered from a psychological disorder tend to have appreciation of beauty, creativity, curiosity, gratitude and love of learning among their top strengths. Those who recover from a serious physical illness have greater appreciation of beauty, bravery, curiosity, fairness, forgiveness, gratitude, humour, kindness, love of learning and spirituality.[6]

Completing a strengths test is one of the most rewarding things you can do for your well-being, both personally and professionally. There are scientific surveys, many of them available online, which will give you the overall picture of your strengths; some of them are general, while others relate more to your work-based strengths.[7] You can take the character strengths test for free at www.viasurvey.org. Allow yourself at least 30 minutes to complete the task and savour the results. Really take the time to appreciate the qualities you have. These are your positive traits.

✦ What are your top five strengths?

✦ Which 'virtues' or categories do your top five belong to?

✦ Are your strengths spread among the virtues or are you dominant in a particular virtue?

✦ What one thing can you do to put each of your top five strengths into action?

There are no right or wrong answers here, this is about getting to know your character strengths and appreciating them for what they give you. I've witnessed transformations as a result of taking a strengths test. On one memorable occasion I was coaching a teenager who was a heavy user of drugs. Danni* had little aspiration, she thought she'd probably end up in prison just like her older brothers. That's what everyone told her. She took the test and discovered that her strengths are predominantly in the virtue of humanity – love, kindness and emotional intelligence. This was no surprise to her, as she was the peacemaker in her family and related well to young children. But having official confirmation of her strengths lit a fire within her. She started attending college regularly,

*Name changed.

she cut back and then gave up the drugs and got herself some work experience. She turned a corner in her life. Having had a pessimistic view of her future, she saw that she didn't have to end up on the same path as her brothers. She now had a goal – to become a youth worker – which was inspiring, played to her strengths and was aligned with her authentic self. As she began to flex her strengths, her confidence soared and life changed. She went through a metamorphosis from teen druggie into a dynamic young woman.

That is an experience of someone who is at the start of their working life. I've also seen the benefits of someone taking a strengths-based approach to changing career in mid-life. Knowing your strengths can clarify your choice of direction and help you to make the change from a more positive perspective with the energy, confidence and motivation to make it happen.

Applying the strong to what's wrong

Your strengths support your psychological well-being and can prevent mental illness. Optimism, for example, protects you against depression and anxiety. Other strengths such as courage, future-mindedness, relationship skills, faith, a work ethic, hope, honesty and perseverance are also known to buffer against mental illness.[8] Using your strengths generates positive emotions and this, in turn, builds resilience so that you're more able to cope with life's trials and bounce back from them.

Your strengths can also help you in therapy. Dr Tayyab Rashid, co-creator of Positive Psychotherapy,[9] recommends that therapists take account of a client's strengths alongside the usual exploration of areas of weakness. This creates a more balanced picture of an individual by highlighting their pluses alongside the minuses, so a client is able to see him- or herself in a more positive light. By having this integrated, holistic understanding of someone, you can see how their strengths might be marshalled to help them undo the troubles that brought them into therapy. Tayyab suggests that therapy clients compose a Positive Introduction – a real-life story that shows them at their best or during a peak moment in their lives, illustrating some of their top strengths in action.

When you're at a low ebb, your strengths can help make things a little easier. Finding ways of using them gives you evidence of things that you *are* good at and boosts your confidence. Your strengths can be applied to build positives and reduce the negatives in life. Here are some coaching activities that will help you make the most of your strengths. This is something that you could do in a coaching session or working with a friend.

A TOOLKIT OF STRENGTHS

Strengths Story: Tell the story of each of your top strengths. When did you first notice that you had this strength? How does it show up in your life now?

→

What are the advantages of having the strength? Discuss situations in which it's been helpful to have this strength. Include examples from your life that illustrate your strengths in action.

Novel Ways to Use Strengths: Brainstorm new ways in which you could apply each of your top five character strengths. Then, commit to some dates on which to try using one or more of your strengths in a new way. Remember that one of the most reliable ways of raising your long-term happiness is to find new ways of using your strengths.

Strengths Solution: Take a real-life issue that you're facing at the moment and see how you might be able to apply each of your top five strengths to find a new way of tackling the problem. This is a good one to do with someone else who may spot things you miss.

Strengths at work

Your strengths are like levers that you can pull to help you achieve your goals. They hold your potential for success in the workplace. The research shows that people who are able to craft their work around their strengths are more engaged in what they do, perform better and enjoy greater success in their roles. People who have the opportunity to focus on their strengths every day are six times more likely to be engaged with their jobs and more than three times as likely to report having an excellent quality of life.[10] It bears repeating that using your strengths in your work is the way to **excel with ease**, because you'll be performing well at something that comes naturally to you. So invest in developing your strengths rather than in fixing your weaknesses. This represents a paradigm shift for the workplace where training is traditionally geared toward developing areas of weakness rather than strength. When you focus on weaknesses there's a ceiling to what you can achieve, because it's something you're not naturally good at. The best you can achieve is mediocrity. But when you focus on developing your strengths, there are no such limits. This is how you are when you're at your strongest and fulfilling your potential. Incidentally, the advice for your areas of weakness is to put in enough effort to master the necessities involved but to channel your efforts instead into your strengths. That is where you will get the best return.

If you're at a crossroads in life, your top strengths will provide you with a strong clue as to which way to move forward. I've seen people turn a corner in their lives when they begin to follow their strengths. It's particularly helpful if you are thinking of embarking on a new career. One of my key strengths is curiosity, which I drew on extensively in an earlier career in the media. Whenever I went to interview someone, my strength of curiosity was brimming with questions at the ready. I carried this strength together with social intelligence, also in my top five, into my work as a psychologist and coach. Curiosity and social intelligence enable me to find out what makes people tick and get to the heart of the matter with speed and ease. Your strengths are like a bundle of talents that you can take from one career into the next, applying them in new ways.

Be aware, though that it is possible to overplay your strengths. Strengths enable high performance, but using them to excess or misapplying them can lead to a loss of performance and things going wrong. That's when you begin to see the shadow side of a strength. Humour overdone can miss its mark or appear as a lack of respect. Leadership taken too far can alienate the people around you. Creativity overdone can lead to many projects started at the expense of projects completed. As we saw with energy, there needs to be some balance between exertion and recovery. Burnout is a risk if the need for renewal is not respected.

The bottom 80

We live in a society that has traditionally rated educational achievement highly and valued it as the path to a happy and thriving life. This narrow definition of success is given to children at an early age, generating anxiety about whether they are good enough to make the grade. One of the beauties of the strengths approach is that it celebrates broader talents beyond academic ones and this is especially important for young people. I've worked with teenagers who've dropped out of education and had zero belief in being good at anything besides a talent for getting into trouble. Helping disaffected young people to identify their strengths builds self-confidence based on something concrete rather than on empty affirmations and gives them a means to reconnect with society. Christine Duvivier, a positive psychologist from Boston, has studied the talents of the 'bottom 80 percent', that is those of the majority rather than the elite.[11] She refutes many of the myths associated with education, such as that being a top student leads to a great life or that not being a 'top student' means that you're not intelligent, hardworking or gifted. Many capabilities that are well-suited to thriving in adulthood are not nurtured within the existing model of education; talents such as entrepreneurial instincts, manual dexterity, the visual eye or the art of persuasion, which is so critical to sales and marketing. The message to take away from this is that many of our strengths may not be recognized early in life and may not even fit the mould of what's conventionally considered to be a strength, but they hold seeds of success that can be developed at any stage of life, whether at the start of working life, in mid-life or in retirement. Your strengths point you toward a fresh new direction, which can sustain you on your journey out of depression.

The ones to read: *Average to A+: Realising Strengths in Yourself And Others* by Alex Linley

Character Strengths and Virtues: A handbook and classification by Chris Peterson and Martin Seligman

CHAPTER 12

Positive Directions: Moving Forward

✦ **What is it?** The 'eudaimonic' side of happiness – playing to your strengths, functioning well and realizing your potential

✦ **Try this for:** The future, life purpose, setting goals and a new chapter after depression

✦ **If you like this, try also:** Strengths (Chapter 11)

In this final chapter I'd like to invite you to make plans for life beyond the lows. One of the characteristics of depression is to look back and ruminate over how things went wrong, how you suffered a setback or trauma, or how life didn't turn out quite the way you planned. You cannot change the past, but you can influence the shape of your future. Maybe the time has come to draw a line under that old chapter and begin anew. Rise like a phoenix from the ashes.

Depression can act as a signal that your current lifestyle is no longer working well for you. It is a sign that something has to change. In my own case it wasn't until I'd experienced several episodes of depression that I finally realized that I was on the wrong career path. Having made the changes I am much happier; I play to my strengths and no longer suffer from the crippling lows that once had me in their grip. The good news is that the past is not necessarily an indicator of the future. You have a high degree of influence over how things turn out and that applies even if you have a high external locus of control, that is you believe your life is ruled by other forces (such as a higher power, fate, karma, other people, the planets, etc). Perhaps it is time now to let go of being a victim of that past difficulty, to move beyond it and to look forward to a future where you operate from a position of strength. There are tools in this chapter to help you move forward positively, in a direction that is right for you now and with a sense of purpose that is authentic to you, aligned to who you really are.

Positive psychology is a science with many different facets but it can be summarized as being about two fundamental things: **how to feel good** and **how to function well**. **Feeling good** is the more familiar side of the field that we've focused on in earlier chapters – it's about experiencing an abundance of positive emotions, the high of happiness and a cheerful mood. **Functioning well** relates to a deeper sense of well-being. It's how we are when we're playing to our strengths, when we're at our best and fulfilling our potential. It's about having meaning and purpose, experiencing personal growth and fulfilment. This is 'eudaimonic' well-being (*see* page 33), which is based on actualizing your true nature or 'daimon'. The original concept of this dates back to the ancient Greek philosophers. It's a 'quieter' form of happiness, which many psychologists think leads to a greater satisfaction with life and a more stable sense of well-being. In this chapter we look at some of the elements that make up this form of well-being and how we can have more of it.

The meaning of life

What gives your life meaning? Is it your loved ones, your faith, your vocation, your achievements? Or is it creative expression or your journey of self-discovery? Whatever the source, it's a deeply personal matter. Big life events lend meaning to life, whether that's something positive, such as the birth of a child, or negative in the case of a trauma. Life is said to be meaningful when it has a significance that goes beyond the momentary or the trivial, or when it has a purpose or coherence that transcends chaos.[1] Whichever the case, those who have a sense of meaning in life have better well-being than those who don't. A lack of meaning is one of the symptoms of depression. My last episode of depression came when I found that the meaning had vanished from my life. Motherhood was the path I wanted to be on, but when it became clear that this was not going to happen (at least in the conventional sense) the door opened to depression. What really helped with recovery was to find a new purpose in life that was meaningful and motivating. My life purpose now is to help people onto the path to happiness and it is every bit as inspiring as when I first articulated it. It brings me great satisfaction when I fulfil my purpose in working with people. It delivers all the meaning in life that I need – and more.

Positive experiences provide us with a sense that things are as they are meant to be. Even simple pleasures can give meaning to life, such as a lazy sunny afternoon spent in the company of a loved one. Equally, some of the most traumatic experiences can lend meaning to your life as you engage in making sense of what has occurred. Viktor Frankl, the Austrian psychiatrist, wrote *Man's Search for Meaning*[2] about the time he spent incarcerated in a Nazi concentration camp. In the midst of his suffering and deprivation, Frankl describes an incident in which he was working in harsh, icy conditions and suddenly had a vision of his wife accompanied by a feeling of bliss. For him the revelation was that love gives life its greatest meaning. Even with nothing left in the world, it was possible to experience meaning. Frankl suggests that meaning is found through these routes:

✦ Creating a work or carrying out a deed.

✦ Experiencing something or encountering someone.

✦ By the attitude we take toward unavoidable suffering.

One of the most potent ways of bringing meaning into your existence is to have a purpose in life, a sense of knowing what you're about and the work you were born to do. Not only does it provide you with two of the three main pathways to happiness – meaning and engagement[3] – but it also gives you a sense of direction, inspiration, motivation and a target for your energy and goals to aim for. Having a purpose gives you a stable bedrock in life, which enables you to be more resilient to stresses and strain. Do you have a sense of your purpose in life? If not, you're not the only one. Many people feel little sense of purpose, wondering what they're meant to be doing with their lives and hesitating between many options, not knowing which to choose. Others doubt that there is a purpose in life for them. The big question is how do you find your purpose in life? Research suggests it comes about in one of three ways.[4]

✦ Being proactive, investing effort over time to clarify your life purpose.

✦ Through a transformative life event such as an illness or parenthood.

✦ Observing others and basing your purpose on what you learn from them.

So your life purpose is something you work toward or it arrives fully-formed or it emerges vicariously through your observation of other people's vocations. It can feel quite daunting to set about identifying something as significant as your purpose in life. Remember to keep a 'growth mindset' (*see* page 21)about it – this is about trial and error, your purpose is not set in stone, but is something that can evolve over time and change throughout your life. There is often a deep sense of knowing when you connect with a purpose that is right for you. It feels congruent. You may experience the body relaxing, breathing out. Trust your gut instinct on this one. Below are some activities that can help you to identify your life purpose, starting with one based on some of your most memorable positive moments.[5] Enjoy!

DISCOVERING YOUR LIFE PURPOSE – 1

Think of **three of the most positive, peak experiences** of your life:

1. ....

....

2. ....

....

3. ....

....

For the first one, ask yourself, '**What was important to me about this experience?**' Outline two reasons for each experience writing a couple of sentences on each. Repeat for the other positive experiences.

→

- ....
  ....

- ....
  ....

- ....
  ....

- ....
  ....

- ....
  ....

- ....
  ....

- When you've finished, underline the keywords in each sentence. These relate to your core values.
- From this list select and **circle the three most important ones** to you.

→

- With these top three in mind, have a go at writing a simple **life purpose** statement. Play around with the order of the words until an idea of your life purpose emerges. Stay in a light mood as you experiment with it and keep going until you formulate a sentence that feels right for you. Have a guess if you're not sure.

My purpose in life is to...

....

....

....

Relax and enjoy the process. There is no right or wrong answer here. Your life purpose can change over time.

This exercise works well because it reveals your purpose in life via an indirect route. I've found it to be a powerful process to use with coaching clients, who often experience light-bulb moments as they formulate their life purpose. Once you've generated a purpose, notice if it is a good fit for you. Does it feel authentic to you and motivating? Having a new (or renewed) life purpose will help to move you forward and is especially useful if you're at a career crossroads. Think of one small, manageable step now that you could take toward living your life purpose. You might do some research on the Internet or make a phone call. Whatever it is put a date in the diary and commit to taking that small step.

Next is another activity that can help you to get closer to identifying your source of meaning and purpose in life. I recommend getting yourself into a resourceful state beforehand to help the process – go for a walk, meditate, listen to music or spend some time in nature. This exercise involves writing, so you might want to use a journal to record your thoughts.

Positive legacy

✦ Think ahead to your life as you would like it to be and how you would prefer to be remembered by the people closest to you.

✦ What would you like them to say about you? What accomplishments and strengths would they mention?

✦ Allow yourself to daydream freely on the subject and give rein to your imagination. Try to keep it grounded in reality rather than being too much of a fantasy. Don't be too modest though – think big.

✦ Write a couple of paragraphs on your positive legacy.

✦ Put it away for a while. When you come to look at it again, notice what the themes are. What does it tell you about what gives meaning to your life? What clues does it give you about your purpose?

✦ Look back at what you've written and ask yourself the following questions: What can I do that is within

my control to bring about my legacy? What am I
currently doing that will move me closer to this goal?

Based on Chris Peterson's *A Primer in Positive Psychology*[6]

Depression is often preceded and precipitated by endings
– a relationship, a job, a stage in life, a way of life. Painful
as that is, once the mourning process is underway, endings also pave the way for new beginnings. Having a goal
is a major step in the recovery from depression, to help
you move forward in a new and positive direction. My
own experience of emerging from depression felt like the
proverbial phoenix rising from the ashes. The old life had
crashed and burned. It was time to find a new direction,
although I tried my best to cling on to my old ways. One
of the things that really helped with building a new life
was to focus on my strengths and to use them to identify
a new direction and then to power the move into the new
area. Your strengths point you toward a life purpose that
is authentic and aligned with who you really are. Here
is another activity to help you to identify your purpose,
based on the strengths that you discovered in the previous chapter.

DISCOVERING YOUR LIFE PURPOSE – 2

Your strengths and other gifts are a clue to your
vocation. Use this exercise to clarify a direction for
applying your strengths.[7]

→

- Write a list of your top five character strengths from the VIA test.

  1. ....

  2. ....

  3. ....

  4. ....

  5. ....

- Write a list of around five other talents/gifts that you have – for example, you are artistic, sporty, musical, good with animals, make people laugh, have an eye for colour, etc.

  1. ....

  2. ....

  3. ....

  4. ....

  5. ....

- Write a list of things that make you angry in modern society (choose something that you might feel strongly enough to act upon).

  1. ....

  →

2. ....

3. ....

Now pick one item from each category – whatever most attracts your attention from each list – and note them below.

a .... b ....

c ....

Use these three elements to formulate a life purpose statement as follows.

I'm going to take my strength in ....

and my gift for ....

to ....

(your anger expressed in the positive, as a call to action)*

Have a go – there is no right or wrong answer. If you don't know, guess!

---

* For example, if your anger is about the extent of mental illness in modern society, your statement expressed as a positive would be 'to promote psychological well-being' rather than 'to stop mental illness'.

Life rewards action

I hope you have more of an understanding now of eudaimonic well-being – the deeper well-being that arises from having meaning and purpose in life alongside a greater knowledge of your personal strengths and how you might draw on them to help you move forward. Depression is a debilitating condition and taking action can be the last thing you feel like doing. However, in order to move beyond being stuck requires you to take action and that is when life will begin to change. So here are some tips that can support you in turning a thought into a deed, which will help to bring about change and live your life purpose.

A nudge in the right direction

+ Aim low not high. Taking many small steps is more likely to get the ball rolling rather than one big step. Set the bar low – foothills rather than mountains.

+ Be kind to yourself and act in the moments when your mood is lighter. This could be after some physical or social activity.

+ Take just one step a day. If there were a mantra to hold in mind it is this: try to do just one small thing to take you forward each day.

Goal-setting for change

Coaching asks one fundamental question – 'What do you want?' This contrasts with 'What is wrong?' the question at the heart of counselling. This next section looks at what you would like for your life beyond the depression. What would you like to achieve? That might seem like an alien concept right now, but having a goal gives you a direction in life, something to aim for, a purpose. And there is quite a bit of research that suggests that satisfaction with life is gained through achieving goals that are important to you. Goal-setting is a mixed bag to someone in depression. Sometimes it is the failure to achieve your life goals that acts as a trigger to depression. This is especially the case in mid-life. Happiness tends to hit a low point in the mid-forties; realizing that it may be too late to achieve certain goals might be a factor in the mid-life crisis. But sometimes giving up on those long-held goals is what finally allows you to move forward. The good news is that after this mid-life dip happiness starts to rise again.[8]

I think it is best with goals to hold them lightly – more as intentions that give you a direction rather than as fixed points that you *must* achieve where the failure to reach them might weigh heavily. My happiness began to rise once I gave up on those long-held ambitions that I hadn't achieved and set intentions that were more flexible and with a greater acceptance of what is. What follows are a series of exercises to help you to get clearer about the direction you want now for your life.

THE WHEEL OF WELL-BEING

This is a simple process to help you to work out which areas of your life need attention and where to focus your efforts to increase your well-being. Draw a circle or a wheel and divide it into eight segments. Label each part with an area of life – below is a list of some of the major areas of well-being, but feel free to include others that are significant for you.

- **Joy** – Fun, leisure and pleasure

- **Meaning** – Purpose, fulfilment, spirituality

- **Connection** – Relationships with loved ones, friends, others

- **Resilience** – Ability to deal with difficulty and bounce back

- **Vitality** – Physical health, energy, exercise

- **Personal Development** – Learning, self-expression

- **Work** – Career satisfaction

- ....

- ....

- ....

See example of Wheel of Well-being overleaf.

Your Wheel of Well-being

Label each section of the wheel with a life area. Then rate
how satisfied you are with each area by drawing a line
within the section. Score each area on a scale from 0 (very
poor) to 10 (very good). The centre of the wheel is 0 and
the outer edge is 10. A high score will place a line near
the outer edge and a low score near the centre.

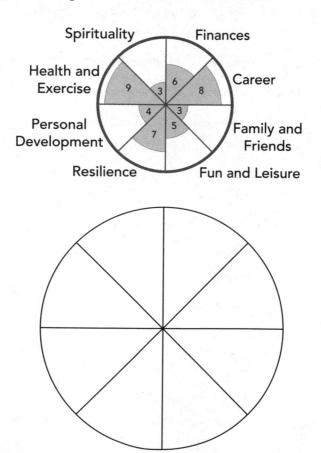

Once you've completed your Wheel of Well-being, ask yourself the following questions.

✦ How do you rate your well-being? What do you notice in your wheel?

✦ What is working well?

✦ What needs attention?

✦ Which part of the wheel can you address first?

✦ What one small step could you take to make a big difference somewhere on your wheel?

Copy each segment over into a Life-planning Chart like the one on page 237. Then, set a goal for each area of life, making sure that you express it as an approach goal, that is, as something you want to move toward rather than an avoidant goal of something you want to get away from. Approach goals are more likely to be intrinsically motivating – something that you want for its own sake. The opposite, extrinsic motivation, is when you are motivated to do something because it will bring you an external reward, such as better status, etc. Having an intrinsically motivating goal is more likely to inspire you to put the effort in and persist when the going gets tough.

Make sure that it is a manageable goal. Think SMART – Specific, Measurable, Attainable, Relevant and with a Time-frame attached. The point of this is that if it is too big a target, the risk is that you might find it too daunting to tackle or give up once you run into obstacles and label yourself as a failure. The secret is to keep the goal small enough to encourage yourself into action. Right now it's about moving off the starting block; you can take bigger steps further down the line when you feel ready for them. Your goal needs to be specific so that you have a real sense of what you're aiming for, such as going to the gym once a week rather than 'to get fit', which is more vague. Identify a first step toward this goal. Make sure it's easy, something that is well within your grasp. And then identify the next step.

With your goal in mind, consider your answer to the following questions, which will help you to further develop your vision for your goal.

+ If I could wave a magic wand and give you your goal right now, would you say yes without hesitation? If in doubt, then you may need to refine the goal further, so that the answer is a confident yes.

+ Get really specific about your goal. What is it you want? When? Where? Who else is involved?

+ How might it come about? Be creative and list as many ways that you can think of. Put to one side any restrictions as you write your list.

+ What resources would help you achieve your goal? People, organizations, books or websites?

+ What will it be like when you achieve your goal? What evidence might you see? What might you hear? What will you feel? Use your senses to imagine how it will be – sights, sounds and feelings.

LIFE-PLANNING CHART

Life area ....

....

SMART Goal ....

....

....

....

First step – make it easy ....

....

....

....

....

Next step ....

....

....

....

....

✦ Is the goal the right size to motivate you to take action? If it is too big, reduce its size to something manageable. If it is too small, set the bar a bit higher so that you feel more inspired.

✦ Notice where you are on the journey to your goal. What progress has already been made?

✦ Adjust your goal, if necessary, to ensure that is based on something within your control.

Here are a couple of questions that can help you to prepare for that first step.

✦ What has to happen for you to achieve your goal?

✦ What's stopping you at the moment from reaching your goal?

The first question will clarify the details of the first step to take, whereas the second question will highlight what obstacles are currently in your way.

Where there's a will, there's a way ...

At this point I'd like to introduce you to Hope, the more retiring cousin of Optimism (*see* Chapter 7). Hope doesn't get the same attention as her more prominent relation, but nonetheless has something valuable to offer to goal-setting. Hope in positive psychology is much more than a belief in a positive outcome, it is a very practical concept. There are two parts to it: firstly, having the motivation to achieve goals (agency); and secondly, having a clear idea of how to get to the goals (pathways).[9] Hopelessness as a feeling is all too common in depression, but even if you don't *feel* hopeful about your goal, what the positive psychology version of hope offers is a concrete strategy to develop hopefulness and move toward your goal. This is the positive psychology recipe for hope:

1. Identify what you want (goals).

2. Think of a variety of routes toward your goal (pathways).

3. Apply yourself with energy to achieving that goal and keep going (agency).

With hope it's a case of where there's a will (agency), there's almost certainly a way (a pathway, in fact). What differentiates hopeful people from non-hopeful people is that when they find an obstacle on their route to a goal, they will be flexible and look for other pathways to reach it. And this is where 'agency' comes into play, giving a hopeful person the energy and motivation to get started on the goal and to persist when the going gets tough. You may find it a struggle to be authentically hopeful, but here is a formula that removes the frustration and instead deconstructs hope into a series of steps that can take you on the way to your goal: from helplessness to hopefulness.

Happily ever after?
The maintenance diet

This book has detailed evidence-based positive psychology techniques that build happiness and well-being, taking you up the mental health scale to a state of flourishing. These strategies can be applied to boost your mood naturally, protect you from the downward spiral into depression and support you in overcoming the 'black dog'. Depression has many varied causes and your recovery will similarly benefit from taking a multi-faceted approach.

✦ Invest in positive emotions to build resilience and reach the positivity ratio.

✦ Practise optimism, the key tool of positive thinking.

✦ Connect to the people in your life for social well-being.

✦ Focus on the physical bedrock of well-being – energy, diet, exercise.

✦ Reflect on the bigger picture – your meaning and purpose in life.

✦ Use your strengths as levers to pull to support you in reaching your goals.

Remember that while pleasure will give you the high of happiness in the moment, there is a deeper well-being that comes from having meaning and purpose in life and being engaged in activities that allow you to realize your potential.

'This too shall pass'

Optimists tend to react to the bad events in their lives by thinking that it is a temporary state of affairs. That 'this too shall pass'. Applying optimism to depression, the good news is that most episodes of depression have a life cycle and will run their course. The recovery from depression can feel like a gradual one – you may not even notice how the dark is receding while the light is increasing by degrees. Slowly and surely there will be more frequent experiences of positive emotion and fewer days in the depths of despair.

The research indicates that once you've had depression, you're at a greater risk of having further episodes, hence the need for a maintenance diet of mood-boosting activities to keep the blues at bay. Look after your mental well-being and give it as much attention as you would your physical well-being. Simple ways you can do that is by savouring the good things as they happen, practising the art of appreciation, reframing the negative and paying attention to the balance in your life between work, rest and play. Remember that around 40 percent of your happiness is under your direct control, so there's a lot that you can influence. Fill your reservoir of well-being with experiences that generate positive emotions or bring meaning into your life. This will build your resilience, help you to sail through life's ups and downs and give you greater protection against depression when you next come to navigate the stormy waters of life.

Learn to recognize the signs that you might be heading into a downward spiral and use that as a cue to augment your practice of the techniques in the book. Apart from the occasional low mood, I now live life free from depression and my capacity for happiness is much greater than it has ever been. Developing that 40 percent made all the difference. The same can happen for you, too. Things are more flexible than they are fixed. Life does change. Every cell in your body will renew itself. What you focus on grows. You can grow your happiness, increase your positivity, learn optimism even if you were a born pessimist and develop your strengths. There is a light at the end of the tunnel even if you don't believe it to be true. There is hope.

'Where there's life, there's hope.' *Cicero*

The one to read: *Creating Your Best Life* by Caroline Adams Miller MAPP and Dr Michael Frisch

Chapter notes

Introduction
1 The Positive Psychology Center at the University of Pennsylvania (www.ppc.sas.upenn.edu)
2 The Penn Resilience Programme www.ppc.sas.upenn.edu/prpsum.htm

Chapter 1
1 Seligman, M.E.P., Rashid, T., and Parks, A.C. (2006). Positive psychotherapy, *American Psychologist*, 61, 774–788
2 Lambert, M.J. (2004). Bergin and Garfield's *Handbook of Psychotherapy and Behaviour Change*. Chichester: Wiley, 5th edition
3 Berk, M. and Parker, G. (2009). The elephant on the couch: side-effects of psychotherapy, *Australian and New Zealand Journal of Psychiatry*, 43, 787–794
4 Akhtar M. & Boniwell, I. (2010). Applying positive psychology to alcohol-misusing adolescents: A group intervention. *Groupwork*, 20 (3), 7–23
5 Sin, N.L., and Lyubomirsky, S. (2009). Enhancing well-being and alleviating depressive symptoms with positive psychology interventions: A practice-friendly meta-analysis. *Journal of Clinical Psychology: In Session*, 65, 467–487. The meta-analysis of 51 interventions with 4,266 individuals revealed that positive psychology interventions significantly enhance well-being (mean *r* = .29) and decrease depressive symptoms (mean *r* =.31).
6 Seligman, M.E.P., Rashid, T., & Parks, A.C. (2006). Positive psychotherapy. *American Psychologist*, 61, 774–788
7 Johnstone, C. (2010), *Find Your Power*, 2nd ed, Permanent Publications

8 www.nhs.uk/Conditions/Depression
9 Dweck, C.S. (2006). *Mindset: The new psychology of success*. New York: Random House

Chapter 2
1 Lyubomirsky, S., Sheldon, K.M., and Schkade, D. (2005). Pursuing happiness: The architecture of sustainable change. *Review of General Psychology*, 9, 111–131
2 Seligman, M.E.P. (2003). *Authentic Happiness* London: Nicholas Brealey Publishing; Lyubomirsky, S.(2007) *The HOW of Happiness*. London: Sphere
3 Seligman, op.cit.
4 Seligman, M.E.P. (2011). *Flourish*. London: Nicholas Brealey Publishing
5 Diener, E. (2000) Subjective Well-being: The science of happiness and a proposal for a national index. *American Psychologist*, 55, 56–67
6 Ryff, C.D. & Keyes, C.L.M. (1995) The structure of psychological well-being revisited. *Journal of Personality and Social Psychology*, 69, 719–727
7 Csikszentmihalyi, M. (1990). *Flow: The Psychology of Optimal Experience*, New York: Harper and Row
8 Ryan, R.M., & Deci, E.L. (2000). Self-determination theory and the facilitation of intrinsic motivation, social development, and well-being. *American Psychologist*, 55, 68–78
9 Mauss, I.B., Tamir, M., Anderson, C.L., and Savino, N.S. (2011). Can seeking happiness make people happy? Paradoxical effects of valuing happiness. *Emotion*, 1–9

Chapter 3
1 Fredrickson, B.L. (2001). The role of positive emotions in positive psychology: The broaden-and-build

theory of positive emotions. *American Psychologist, 56*, 218–26

2 Fredrickson, B.L. (2009). *Positivity.* New York: Crown Publishers

3 Fredrickson B.L. & Losada M.F. (2005). Positive affect and the complex dynamics of human flourishing. *American Psychologist, 60*, 678–86

4 Schwartz, R.M., Reynolds, C.F., III, Thase, M.E., Frank, E., Fasiczka, A.L., and Haaga, D.A.F. (2002). Optimal and normal affect balance in psychotherapy of major depression: Evaluation of the balanced states of mind model. *Behavioural and Cognitive Psychotherapy, 30*, 439–50

5 Lyubomirsky, S., King, L.A., and Diener, E. (2005). The benefits of frequent positive affect. *Psychological Bulletin, 131*, 803–55

6 Frisch, M.B. (2006). *Quality of Life Therapy.* New Jersey: John Wiley & Sons

Chapter 4

1 Bryant, F.B. & Veroff, J. (2007). *Savoring: A new model of positive experiences.* Mahwah, N.J., Lawrence Erlbaum Associates, Inc.

2 Honoré, C. (2005). *In Praise of Slow: How a Worldwide Movement is Challenging the Cult of Speed.* London: Orion Books

3 www.slowfood.com

4 Schooler, J.W., Ariely, D., & Loewenstein, G. (2003). The pursuit and assessment of happiness may be self-defeating. In I. Brocas & J.D. Carilloo (eds). *The psychology of economic decisions. Volume 1: Rationality and well-being* (pp.41–70) New York: Oxford University Press

5 Bryant & Veroff, op cit.

6 Diener, Sanvik & Pavot (1991). Happiness is the frequency, not the intensity of positive versus negative affect. In F. Strack, M. Argyle, & N. Schwarz (eds.), *Subjective well-being: An interdisciplinary perspective* (pp.119–139). New York: Pergamon

7 Seligman, M.E.P, Rashid, T. & Parks, A.C. (2006) Positive psychotherapy. *American Psychologist 61*, pp.774–88

8 Boniwell, I., & Zimbardo, P. (2004). Balancing time perspective in pursuit of optimal functioning. In P.A. Linley & S. Joseph (eds.), *Positive psychology in practice.* New Jersey: John Wiley & Sons

9 Bryant, F.B., Smart, C.M., & King, S.P. (2005). Using the past to enhance the present: Boosting happiness through positive reminiscence. *Journal of Happiness Studies, 6*, 227–60

Chapter 5

1 Breathnach, S.B. (1996). *The simple abundance journal of gratitude.* New York: Warner

2 Lyubomirsky, S. (2007). *The HOW of Happiness.* London: Sphere Books

3 Emmons, R. (2007) *Thanks! How the new science of gratitude can make you happier,* Boston: Houghton Mifflan Company

4 Lyubomirsky, S. (2007), op cit., p.91

5 Emmons, R. op.cit.

6 Pollay, D.J. (2008) Gratitude is a bridge to your positive future. Retrieved at positivepsychologynews.com/news/david-j-pollay/200811021119

7 Gratitude: How to appreciate life's gifts (2010). *Positive Psychology News Series*

8 Emmons, R.A. & Shelton, C.M. (2005). Gratitude and the Science of Positive Psychology. In C.R. Snyder & S.J. Lopez (eds.), *Handbook of Positive Psychology* (pp.459–71). London: Oxford University Press

9 Seligman, M.E.P., Steen, T.A., Park, N., & Peterson, C. (2005). Positive psychology progress: Empirical

validation of interventions. *American Psychologist*, 60, 410–21

10 Ibid.

11 For more on Appreciative Inquiry: Cooperrider, D.L., and Whitney, D. (2005). *Appreciative Inquiry: A positive revolution in change*. San Francisco: Berrett-Koehler Publishers

Chapter 6

1 Kabat-Zinn, J. (1994). *Mindfulness Meditation for Everyday Life*. Piatkus Books

2 Davidson, R.J., Kabat-Zinn, J., Schumacher, J., Rosenkranz, M., Muller, D., Santorelli, S.F., et al. (2003). Alterations in brain and immune function produced by mindfulness meditation. *Psychosomatic Medicine*, 65, 564–70

3 Find out more about Prof Richard Davidson's work in the Lab for Affective Neuroscience at http://psyphz.psych.wisc.edu/

4 Shapiro, S.L., Schwartz, G.E.R. & Santerre, C. (2005). Meditation and positive psychology. In C.R. Snyder & S.J. Lopez (eds.), *Handbook of positive psychology* (pp.632–645). London: Oxford University Press

5 Fredrickson, B., Cohn, M., Coffey, K. A, Pek, J., & Finkel, S.M. (2008). Open hearts build lives: Positive emotions induced through loving-kindness meditation, build consequential personal resources. *Journal of Personality and Social Psychology*, 95 (5), 1045–1062

6 The Buddhist Education and Information Network has guidance on loving-kindness and other meditations at www.buddhanet.net

7 Williams, M., Teasdale, J., Segal, Z. & Kabat-Zinn, J. (2007). *The mindful way through depression: Freeing yourself from chronic unhappiness*. New York: Guilford Press

8 Hanh, T.N. (1991). *The Miracle of Mindfulness*. London: Rider Books

9 Davidson, Kabat-Zinn, Schumacher, Rosenkranz, Muller, Santorelli et al. Op cit.

10 Kabat-Zinn, J. (1990). *Full Catastrophe Living: Using the wisdom of your body and mind to face stress, pain and illness*. New York: Delacorte Press

11 Reibel, D.K., Greeson, J.M., Brainard, G.C., et al (2001). Mindfulness-based stress reduction and health-related quality of life in a heterogeneous patient population. *General Hospital Psychiatry, 23*, 183–92

12 Segal, Z., Teasdale, J., Williams, M. (2002). *Mindfulness-Based Cognitive Therapy for Depression*. New York: Guilford Press

13 Williams, Teasdale, Segal & Kabat-Zinn. Op cit.

Chapter 7

1 Carver, C.S., Scheier, M.F. & Segerstrom, S.C. (2010). Optimism. *Clinical Psychology Review*. 879–889

2 Seligman, M.E.P. (1990). *Learned Optimism*. New York: Knopf

3 Boniwell, I. (2006). *Positive Psychology in a Nutshell*. London: PWBC.

4 Isaacowitz, D.M. & Seligman, M.E.P. (2001) Is pessimism a risk factor for depressive mood among community-dwelling older adults? *Behaviour Research and Therapy, 39*, 255–272.

5 Norem, J.K. (2001). *The Positive Power of Negative Thinking*. New York: Basic Books.

6 Seligman. op cit.

7 Nolen-Hoeksema, S. (1990). *Sex differences in depression*. Stanford, CA: Stanford University Press.

8 Frisch, M.B. (2006). *Quality of Life Therapy*. New Jersey: John Wiley & Sons

9 King, L.A. (2001). The health benefits

of writing about life goals. *Personality and Social Psychology Bulletin*, 27, 798–807.

10 Sheldon, K. M., & Lyubomirsky, S. (2006). How to increase and sustain positive emotion: The effects of express expressing gratitude and visualizing best possible selves, *The Journal of Positive Psychology*. 1(2), 73–82.

11 Schneider, S.L. (2001). In search of realistic optimism. *American Psychologist*, 56(3), 250–263.

12 Segerstrom, S.C. (2006). *Breaking Murphy's Law*. New York: Guilford

Chapter 8

1 This description of resilience comes from Dr Chris Johnstone in *Find Your Power*, 2010, Permanent Publications

2 Masten, A.S. (2001). Ordinary magic: Resilience processes in development. *American Psychologist*, 56, 227–38

3 Reivich, K & Shatté, A. (2002). *The Resilience Factor*. New York: Broadway Books

4 Carr, A. (2004). *Positive Psychology*. Hove: Brunner-Routledge

5 Based on Zeidner, M. & Endler, N. S. (eds.) (1996). *Handbook of Coping: Theory, Research, Applications*. New York: John Wiley

6 Both *The Optimistic Child* by Martin Seligman et al and *The Resilience Factor* by Karen Reivich and Andrew Shatté explore the ABC Model in detail.

7 Reivich, K. and Shatté, A. (2002). *The Resilience Factor*. New York: Broadway Books

8 Based on Burns, D.D. (1980). *Feeling Good: The New Mood Therapy* (preface by Aaron T. Beck). New York: William Morrow and Co

9 Tugade, M. & Fredrickson, B.L. (2004). Resilient individuals use positive emotions to bounce back from negative emotional

experiences. *Journal of Personality and Social Psychology*, 86 (2), 320–33

10 Fredrickson, B.L. (2009). *Positivity*. New York: Crown Publishers

11 www.depressionalliance.org/

12 Tennen, H. & Affleck, G. (2005). Benefit-Finding and Benefit-Reminding. In C.R. Snyder & S.J. Lopez (eds). *The Handbook of Positive Psychology*. New York: Oxford University Press

13 Tedeschi, R.G., & Calhoun, L.G. (2004). A clinical approach to post-traumatic growth. In P.A. Linley & S. Joseph (eds.), *Positive Psychology in Practice* (pp.405–19). Hoboken, N.J., John Wiley & Sons

14 Based on Nolen-Hoeksema, S. and Davis, C.G. (2005). Positive Responses to Loss. In C.R. Snyder & S.J. Lopez (eds). *The Handbook of Positive Psychology*. New York: Oxford University Press

15 For more on post-traumatic growth. Hefferon, K., Grealy, M., & Mutrie, N. (2009). Post-traumatic growth and life threatening physical illness: a systematic review of the qualitative literature. *British Journal of Health Psychology*, 14 (2), 343–78

16 Niederhoffer, K.G. & Pennebaker, J.W. (2005). Sharing one's story. In C.R. Snyder and S.J. Lopez (eds). *The Handbook of Positive Psychology*. New York: Oxford University Press

17 Pennebaker, J.W. (1989). Confession, inhibition and disease. In L. Berkowitz (ed.), *Advances in experimental social psychology*, 22, 211–44. New York: Academic Press

Chapter 9

1 Chris Peterson, author of *A Primer in Positive Psychology* (2006, NY: Oxford University Press), says that positive psychology can be summed up in three words – 'other people matter'.

2 Diener, E., & Seligman, M.E.P. (2002). Very happy people. *Psychological Science, 13,* 81–84

3 Seligman, M.E.P (1995). *The Optimistic Child.* New York: Houghton Mifflin

4 www.gottman.com

5 Gottman, J.M. & Silver, N. (1999). *The Seven Principles for Making Marriage Work.* New York: Crown Publishers

6 Gable, S.L., Reis, H.T., Impett, E., & Asher, E.R. (2004). What do you do when things go right? The intrapersonal and interpersonal benefits of sharing positive events. *Journal of Personality and Social Psychology, 87,* 228–45

7 Ibid.

8 Goleman, D. (2006). *Social Intelligence: The New Science of Human Relationships.* New York: Bantam Books

9 Kathryn Britton's ideas on social contagion are at: positive psychologynews.com/news/ kathryn-britton/20080407704

10 Dutton, J. (2003). *Energize Your Workplace: How to Create and Sustain High-Quality Connections at Work.* San Francisco, CA: Jossey-Bass

11 Festinger, L. (1954). A theory of social comparison processes. *Human Relations, 7* (2) 117–140

12 Fredrickson, B. (2009). *Positivity: Groundbreaking Research Reveals How to Embrace the Hidden Strength of Positive Emotions, Overcome Negativity, and Thrive.* New York: Crown

13 Bryant, F.B. & Veroff, J. (2007). *Savoring: A new model of positive experiences.* Mahwah, N.J., Lawrence Erlbaum Associates, Inc.

14 Lyubomirsky, S. (2007). *The HOW of Happiness.* London: Sphere Books

15 Weinstein, N. and Ryan, R. (2010). When helping helps: Autonomous motivation for pro-social behaviour and its influence on well-being for the helper and recipient. *Journal of Personality and Social Psychology, 98* (2), 222–44

16 Here are some resources to get you started on spreading kindness: www.randomactsofkindness.org www.thekindnessoffensive.com www.payitforwardfoundation.org

17 McCullough, M.E and van Oyen Witvliet, C. (2005). The Psychology of Forgiveness. In C.R. Snyder & S.J. Lopez (eds). *The Handbook of Positive Psychology.* New York: Oxford University Press

18 Read inspiring stories of forgiveness at www.theforgivenessproject.com

19 I can recommend *The Facebook Manager* (Management Books, 2009) by Bridget Grenville-Cleave and Jonathan Passmore on the psychology and practice of social networking

20 Dunbar, R. (2010) *How Many Friends Does One Person Need? Dunbar's Number and Other Evolutionary Quirks.* London: Faber

21 Granovetter, M. (1983). The strength of weak ties: A network theory revisited. *Sociological Theory,* 201–33

22 Canine Charter for Human Health (2008). Retrieved from www. dogstrust.org.uk

23 Nagasawa, M. et al. (2009). 'Dog's Gaze at Its Owner Increases Owner's Urinary Oxytocin During Social Interaction,' *Hormones and Behaviour, 55* (3), 434–41

Chapter 10

1 Babyak M. Blumenthal J.A., Herman S. Khatri P., Doraiswamy M., Moore K., Craighead W.E., Baldewicz T. T., Krishnan K.R. (2000). Exercise treatment for major depression: maintenance of therapeutic benefit at 10 months. *Psychosom Med.* 62: 633–8

2 Barton J. and Pretty J. (2010). What is the best dose of nature and green

exercise for mental health? A meta-study analysis. *Environmental Sci & Tech*, 44 (10), pp. 3947–955

3 Loehr, J. & Schwartz, T. (2003). *The Power of Full Engagement: Managing Energy, Not Time, Is the Key to High Performance and Personal Renewal.* New York: Free Press

Chapter 11

1 Linley, A. (2008). *Average to A+.* Coventry: CAPP Press

2 Clifton, D.O. & Anderson, E.C. (2002). *Strengthsquest.* Washington: The Gallup Organisation & Peterson, Christopher; Seligman, Martin E.P. (2004). *Character Strengths and Virtues: A handbook and classification.* Oxford: Oxford University Press

3 Seligman, M.E.P., Steen, T.A., Park, N. & Peterson, C. (2005). Positive Psychology Progress: Empirical validation of interventions. *American Psychologist*, 60, 410–21

4 Linley, A., Willars, J., Biswas-Diener, R. (2010). *The Strengths Book.* Coventry: CAPP Press

5 Peterson, Christopher; Seligman, Martin E.P. (2004). *Character strengths and virtues: A handbook and classification.* Oxford: Oxford University Press

6 Peterson, C., Park, N., & Seligman, M.E.P. (2006). Greater strengths of character and recovery from illness. *The Journal of Positive Psychology*, 1, 17–26

7 Strengths tests include the VIA (Values in Action Classification of Character Strengths; Peterson & Seligman, 2004) available at www.viacharacter.org; Realise 2 Personality Strengths Project (CAPP, 2010) can be accessed at www.strengths2020.com and Gallup's StrengthsFinder (Hodges & Clifton, 2004) is available via Gallup books and www.strengthsfinder.com

8 Seligman, M.E.P. (2002). Positive psychology, positive prevention, and positive therapy. In C.R. Snyder & S.J. Lopez (eds.), *Handbook of Positive Psychology* (pp. 3–9). New York: Oxford University Press

9 Seligman, M.E.P., Rashid, T., Parks, A.C. (2006). Positive Psychotherapy. *American Psychologist*, 61: 744–88.

10 Rath, T. (2007). *Strengthsfinder 2.0.* New York, The Gallup Organization

11 Read about Christine Duvivier's inspiring work – Appreciating Beauty in the Bottom 80 – at www.christineduvivier.com

Chapter 12

1 Hicks, J.A, & King, L.A. (2009). Meaning in life as a subjective judgment and lived experience. *Social and Personality Psychology Compass*, 3, 638–53

2 Frankl, V.E. (1963). *Man's Search for Meaning.* New York: Simon & Schuster

3 Seligman, M.E.P. (2002). *Authentic Happiness.* New York: Free Press

4 Kashdan, T.B., and McKnight, P. E. (2009). Origins of purpose in life: Refining our understanding of a life well lived. *Psychological Topics*, 18(2), 303–16

5 This exercise is based on one from Neuro-Linguistic Programming

6 Peterson, C., (2006). *A Primer in Positive Psychology.* New York: Oxford University Press

7 I first came across a version of this activity through Neil Crofts, author of *Authentic, How to Make a Living by Being Yourself.* Capstone Press

8 The U-bend of life. Why, beyond middle age, people get happier as they get older. *The Economist*, Dec 16th 2010

9 Snyder, C.R., Rand, K.L. & Sigmon, D.R. (2005). Hope Theory. In Snyder, C.R., & Lopez, S.J. (eds) *Handbook of Positive psychology.* London: Oxford University Press